PHARMACOLOGY - RESEARCH, SAFETY TESTING AND REGULATION

PROPRANOLOL

MEDICAL USES, MECHANISMS OF ACTION AND POTENTIAL ADVERSE EFFECTS

PHARMACOLOGY - RESEARCH, SAFETY TESTING AND REGULATION

Additional books in this series can be found on Nova's website under the Series tab.

Additional e-books in this series can be found on Nova's website under the e-book tab.

PHARMACOLOGY - RESEARCH, SAFETY TESTING AND REGULATION

PROPRANOLOL

MEDICAL USES, MECHANISMS OF ACTION AND POTENTIAL ADVERSE EFFECTS

MISLAV PULJEVIĆ, MD, PHD
EDITOR

New York

Library of Congress Cataloging-in-Publication Data

ISBN: 978-1-63482-974-8
Library of Congress Control Number: 2015940242

Published by Nova Science Publishers, Inc. † New York

Contents

Preface

Why to write a book about one outdated medicine, about first clinically significant beta blocker? Propranolol is in medical practice since 1962. and still has important role in treatment of various diseases. Although the cardiovascular system is the main target, it has also important role in neurology, endocrinology, psychiatry and gastroenterology. Unfortunately propranolol is in cardiology unfairly forgotten and defeated due to a fact that recent studies examine only new selective beta blockers. We strongly believe it could be useful to conduct new studies with main focus on propranolol which possibly has more beneficial effect on the survival of patients than selective beta blockers in some cases. However, every now and then there is situation where all other "modern" medicines didn't work, but propranolol did. Moreover there are multiple case reports with new interesting indications where propranolol proved its efficiency.

In this book we will see all benefits of propranolol in mentioned medical branches. Authors of these chapters are elected, distinguished experts in their field of medicine from all over the world. It was great pleasure of mine to have ability of gathering their influential and respectable point of view about this unjustly neglected medication. Moreover chemical theory of propranolol and possible advance of molecule in future are also deliberated. The main idea was to wake knowledge about universality of propranolol, and not to allow to fall into oblivion superseded by modern drugs.

I would like to thank all of the authors who have invested their time and expertise to help make this book possible.

Lastly, I would like to dedicate this book to my beautiful wife Vlatka and my beloved children Rita and Domagoj, who have all selflessly supported me throughout this endeavor.

Editor in chief

Mislav Puljevic, MD, PhD

In: Propranolol
Editor: Mislav Puljević

ISBN: 978-1-63482-974-8

Chapter 1

Propranolol Pharmacology

***Eugen Javor*[1] *and Marko Skelin*[2,•]**
[1]University Hospital Centre Sisters of Mercy, Zagreb, Croatia
[2]General Hospital Sibenik, Medicinal Products' Safety Committee, Croatia

Abstract

The first discovered beta-blocker was pronethanol in 1962, but it was replaced with propranolol, which had a much higher potency and a safer profile. Thus, propranolol became a widely used drug in the treatment of many cardiovascular diseases. Nowadays, because of the non-selective beta-AR blockade, propranolol is not used in the treatment of cardiovascular diseases as much as before. But it is still widely used in the treatment of essential tremor, thyrotoxicosis, thyrotoxic crisis, proliferating IH requiring systemic therapy. It is also used as a prophylaxis for upper gastrointestinal bleedings in patients with portal hypertension and esophageal varices. This chapter reviews the basic pharmacology of propranolol. A brief review of the autonomic nervous systems and physiological effects of catecholamines binding on alpha-AR and beta-AR are included, as an introduction to propranolol pharmacodynamics. Propranolol decreases the chronotropic, inotropic, dromotropic and bathmotropic, and lusitropic response to the beta-AR stimulation. It also increases the plasma renin activity, suppresses lipolysis, glycogenolysis and gluconeogenesis. It reduces the tremor of the extremities, decreases production of aqueous humor and also exerts a quinidine-like membrane action, but at dosages greater than required for the beta-blockade. The exact mechanism of the antihypertensive, antitremor and antimigraine effect of propranolol is still uncertain, however, there are several assumptions regarding mechanisms that may contribute to clinical effects.

This chapter also presents the absorption, distribution, metabolism and elimination of propranolol, including particularities as first-pass metabolism in the liver. In addition, the review of all factors entering pharmacodynamic and pharmacokinetic interactions with propranolol is included.

Keywords: Propranolol, pharmacology, pharmacodynamics, pharmacokinetics

• E-mail: markoskelin@yahoo.com.

Introduction

There are three major types of adrenergic receptors: $alpha_1$, $alpha_2$, and beta. Each of them is divided into three subtypes. The International Union of Basic and Clinical Pharmacology (IUPHAR) classification of adrenergic receptors is presented in Figure 1. [1] It was discovered that the beta-adrenergic receptor (beta-AR) has a novel atypical beta-adrenergic subtype, the putative $beta_4$-AR. The $beta_4$-AR is considered as a low affinity state of the $beta_1$-AR, which awaits genetic and pharmacologic characterization. [2] Norepinephrine, also known as noradrenalin (NR), is released as a neurotransmitter from most sympathetic postganglionic fibers, and as a hormone (into the blood) from adrenal medulla (~20% adrenal medulla secretion). Epinephrine, also known as adrenalin (ADR), is on the other hand released as a hormone from adrenal medulla (~80% of secretion). NR and ADR both stimulate the $alpha_1$, $alpha_2$ and $beta_1$ adrenergic receptors, but only ADR stimulates the $beta_2$-AR. The circulating catecholamines (i.e., norepinephrine, epinephrine) are deactivated by the catechol-O-methyltransferase (COMT) in the liver. The rest of NR, that is located in the neuroeffector junction, is taken into the sympathetic nerve that released it and metabolized intraneuronally by the enzyme monoamine oxidase (MAO). [3]

The AR influences the activity of most tissues and organ systems in the body. Locations and effects of AR are presented in Table 1, while the beta-AR subtype differences are presented in Table 2. [1, 4, 5] The first discovered beta-blocker was pronethanol in 1962. However, it never came into widespread clinical use and was replaced by propranolol, which had a much higher potency and a safer profile.

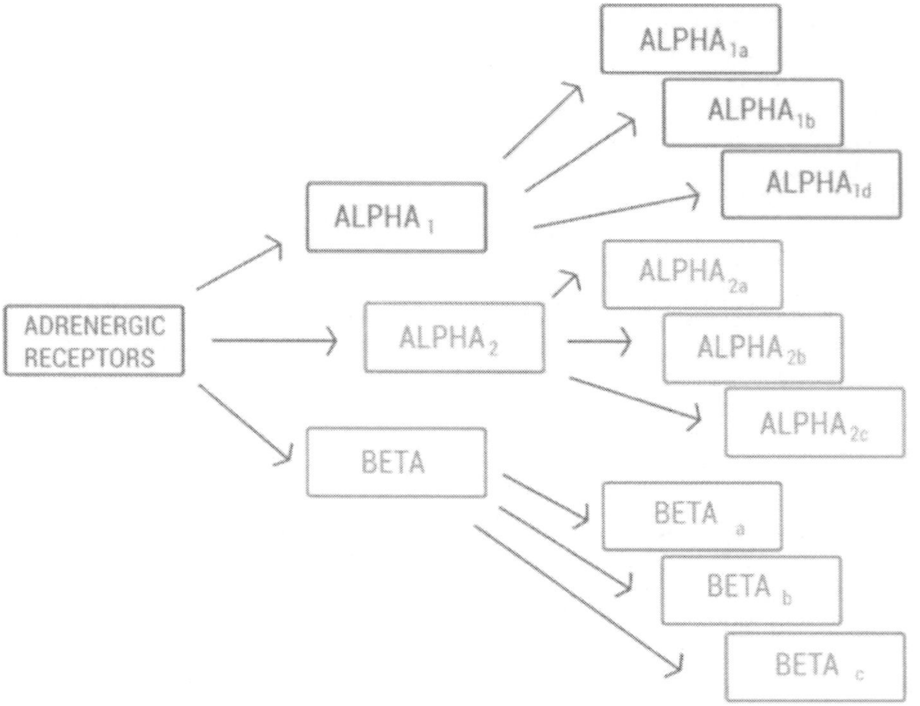

Figure 1. IUPHAR classification of adrenergic receptors.

Table 1. Effects of adrenergic receptors stimulation

Organ	Receptor location	Receptor	Effect
Heart	Sinus node Atria AV node His-Purkinje Ventricle	$\beta_1\ \beta_2$ $\beta_1\ \beta_2$ $\beta_1\ \beta_2$ $\beta_1>\beta_2$ $\beta_1>\beta_2$	Heart rate increase Increase in contractility and conduction velocity AV conduction velocity increase Automaticity increase Increase in contractility and conduction velocity
Vessels	Vessels Arterioles and veins Coronary arteries	$\beta_1\ \beta_2$ β_2 β_1	Constriction Relaxation Relaxation
Lung		β_2	Bronchial muscle relaxation
Skeletal muscle		β_2	Na^+/K^+ jump stimulation, hypokalemia, tremor Increased contractility
Genitourinary tract	Detrusor Bladder sphincter Uterus Sex organ, male	β_2 α_1 β_2 α_1 α_1	Relaxation Contraction Relaxation Contraction Ejaculation
Skin	Pilomotor muscle Sweat glands	α_1 α_2	Contraction Localized secretion
Liver		$\alpha_1\ \alpha_2\ \beta_1$	Glycogenolysis, gluconeogenesis
Intestine	Motility and tone Sphincter Secretion Fat cells Salivary glands	$\alpha_1\ \alpha_2\ \beta_1\ \beta_2$ α_1 α_2 $\alpha_2\ \beta_1$ α_1 β	Decrease Contraction Inhibition Lipolysis K^+ and water secretion Amylase secretion
Eye		β_1 $\beta_1\ \beta_2$	Radial muscle (mydriasis) Intraocular pressure

Abbreviations: AV (atrioventricular), K^+(potassium), Na^+(sodium).

Table 2. Beta adrenergic receptors subtypes differences

Adrenergic receptor	$beta_1$	$beta_2$	$beta_3$
Number of amino acids	477	413	408
Chromosome number	10	5	8
Phosphorylation by PKA and beta-ARK	Yes	Yes	No
Most potent catecholamine	NR	ADR	NR
Selective agonist	Xamoterol Dobutamine	Zinterol Procaterol	BLR 37344 CGP 12177
Selective antagonist	CGP 20712A Metoprolol	ICI 118551	SR 59230A
G-protein	Gs	Gs/Gi	Gs/Gi
Effector	Adenylyl cyclase	Adenylyl cyclase	Adenylyl cyclase NO synthase
Signals	cAMP/PKA	cAMP/PKA MPKA	cAMP/PKA
Tissue receptor location	Heart	Lung Heart Vessels Kidney	Adipose tissue Heart

Abbreviations: PKA (protein kinase A), beta-ARK (beta-adrenergic receptor kinase),NO (nitric oxide), cAMP (cyclic adenosine monophosphate), MPKA (mitogen-activated protein kinase).

It was officially launched in 1964, under the trade name Inderal. Most of the pioneer work in the angina pectoris treatment was done with propranolol, which soon became a widely used drug in the treatment of many cardiovascular diseases. [6, 7] After decades of use, due to the non-selective beta-AR blockade, propranolol slightly lost its place by selective beta-blockers in treatment of cardiovascular diseases.

Pharmacodynamics of Propranolol

As all other beta-blockers, propranolol has a similar chemical structure to endogenous catecholamines, an aromatic cycle, a short lateral chain with an amino function and a hydroxyl group of an alcoholic function. [1] Propranolol is a non-selective competitive antagonist of the beta-AR. *In vitro* propranolol demonstrated a higher selectivity to $beta_2$-AR versus $beta_1$-AR and $beta_3$-AR, 8.3 fold and 141.3 fold, respectively. While comparing selectivity to $beta_1$-AR versus $beta_3$-AR, it was 17.0 fold more selective to $beta_1$-AR. [8]

Propranolol binds reversibly, has no intrinsic sympathomimetic activity, and the associated vasodilating properties. [1, 9] Propranolol is also a 5-hydroxytryptamine$_{1A}$ (5-HT$_{1A}$) antagonist. However, it displays a 50 fold higher affinity for beta-AR than 5-HT$_{1A}$ receptors, and therefore it has a limited utility for *in vivo* studies as a 5-HT$_{1A}$ antagonist. In addition, propranolol binds to 5-HT$_{1B}$ as well. [10] Propranolol is a racemic mixture of equal amounts of S (-) and R (+) isomers. [11] The propranolol S (-) enantiomer is approximately 100 times more potent than the R (+) enantiomer, and is considered as an active form. [12] The R (+) enantiomer has only one additional ancillary property versus the racemic mixture, and that is an inhibition of conversion thyroxine (T4) to triiodothyronine (T3). [13]

Fagan and associates demonstrated that oral propranolol is more effective in lowering the blood pressure than the intravenous (IV) administration (10% vs. 3-5%), and also the IV administration increased the peripheral resistance by 23%, while oral administration had not. [14]

Propranolol was administered in incremental doses of 10, 20, 40, 60, 80, and 120 mg orally, four times a day (q.i.d.), to eight patients with essential hypertension. The heart rate was reduced during rest, tilt and exercise. The blockade of control tachycardia was greater with higher doses, therefore it is dose depended. The cardiac output reduction was also seen with propranolol. [15] Isoproterenol is a non-selective beta-AR agonist with a very low affinity for alpha-AR, and thus exerts positive chronotropic and inotropic effects. It also decreases the peripheral vascular resistance. [16] Propranolol demonstrated a decrease in chronotropic, inotropic, and peripheral vascular responses to isoproterenol. During propranolol treatments, doses of isoproterenol that were required to achieve the same pharmacological effect as without propranolol were 21.9 (chronotropic), 25.0 (inotropic), and 84.8 (vascular) fold higher, respectively. Propranolol reduced the systolic blood pressure during maximal exercise, but only a small hypotensive response was present at rest. These effects can occur after a single oral dose, while multiple dosing may define the blood concentration and a pharmacodynamic relationship with the chronic therapy more accurately. [15] Propranolol decreases the vasodilator responses to the beta-AR stimulation. [17] In anaesthetized dogs, it also reduced the pressor response to NR, but it did not affect the response to phenylephrine. [18] In anaesthetized cats, propranolol did not affect bradycardia, produced by the stimulation of the peripheral end of the right vagus nerve, but it has antagonized the tachycardia completely, produced by the stimulation of the right stellate ganglion. [17]

A negative chronotropic effect of propranolol is the consequence of the competitive antagonism with NR for the beta$_1$-AR. [1] The increase in NR is documented during moderate to severe exercises, and this may explain that propranolol caused a greater reduction in heart rate during exercise than rest. [15]

A negative inotropic effect, seen with propranolol, is mainly due to a blockade of the beta$_1$-AR. However, the beta$_2$-AR is also present in the ventricles and atria, where it also contributes to the cardiac positive inotropic responses. For comparison, the beta$_1$-AR and beta$_2$-AR exist in a 2 vs. 1 ratio in the ventricles and atria. [4] A negative inotropic effect causes a reduction in the cardiac contractile force, systolic ejection volume, and left ventricular ejection fraction. Reduced cardiac outputs and blood pressure are due to a combination of heart rate reductions and a negative inotropic effect. [1] Colin and associates demonstrated on mongrel dogs that the contractility and heart rate both contribute to the myocardial oxygen consumption. [19] Propranolol reduced the myocardial oxygen consumption, aortic blood pressure, and myocardial blood flow on healthy young subjects during exercise. Reduced oxygen requirements are due to a decreasement of the heart rate, systolic blood pressure and the velocity and extent of the myocardial contraction. [20, 21] *Propranolol exerts negative dromotropic effects on the atrioventricular node (AV). It prolongs the atrium to His bundle interval and the AV nodal refractory periods, and it may lengthen the PR interval on an electrocardiogram. [22] It also exerts negative bathmotropic effects, due to a reduction of a refractory period inhomogeneity of Purkinje and myocyte fibers, and a reduction in calcium (Ca2+) overload.* [1] Lucchesi and associates documented in dogs that, reversing or preventing several types of experimentally induced cardiac arrhythmias, is effective with propranolol. [23] Thus, propranolol has a unique importance in managing arrhythmias caused by increased levels of cateholamines, or conditions with enhanced sensitivity of the heart to cateholamines (i.e., pheochromocytoma, thyrotoxicosis, exercise). [21]

The protein kinase C (PKC) activation mediates a sodium/hydrogen (Na^+/H^+) exchanger, induced intracellular alkalosis that accounts for the negative lusitropism of the alpha$_1$-AR stimulation. [24] *In vitro* propranolol changed the phenylephrine-induced positive lusitropic effect, into a negative lusitropic action. [25]

Using the rat left atria S (–) enantiomer (concentration 10^{-8} M) and R (+) enantiomer, (concentration 10^{-6} M) demonstrated a membrane stabilizing activity (sodium Na^+ channel blocking action), due to the inhibition of the responses to an electrical stimulation. [26] *In vitro* within the human muscle, propranolol also demonstrated a membrane stabilizing activity (quinidine-like), but at the minimal concentration of 10 mg/l. In contrast, the concentration required for inhibition of exercise tachycardia or suppression of ectopic beats, is 100 times lower. [27] Therefore, it is not a clinically important property of propranolol.

Propranolol has a cardioprotective effect. It demonstrated an enhanced post-ischaemic recovery of the contractile function. It also demonstrated the suppression of the left ventricular end-diastolic pressure (LVEDP) of the ischaemic/reperfused heart, in a concentration-dependent manner. The study has been conducted in the hearts of rats. Propranolol also blocked the release of the creatine kinase (CK) in a concentration-depended manner, which is a marker of cell necrosis. The cardioprotective effect is probably due to the blocking of Na^+ channels, which are consequently preventing a Na^+ overload in cardiac cells. Excessive Na^+ deteriorates the ATP-generating activity of mitochondria and leads to a reduction of the energy production of the heart during reperfusion. Unfortunately, propranolol was used in largely enhanced concentrations (10 -100 μM), while its clinical relevant concentrations are ~1 μM. [28] Considering the coronary blood flow, propranolol demonstrated no significant change. [29]

Propranolol may produce cold extremities, could favor incidences of Raynaud's phenomenon, and cause or worsen the symptoms of the intermittent claudication. It would happen by causing a drop in the cardiac output or by directly blocking the beta$_2$-AR. [9,30] However, there is not enough evidence to suggest that propranolol adversely affects walking distances, calf blood flows, calf vascular resistances and skin temperatures in patients with intermittent claudication. [31]

The decrease in the cardiac output (negative chronotropic and inotropic effects) decrease in renin, angiotensin II and aldosterone concentrations. The diminution of tonic sympathetic nerve outflow from vasomotor centers in the brain all contribute to lowering the blood pressure. [15, 32, 33] Assumptions exist that propranolol may achieve a better antihypertensive effect in patients with normal or elevated plasma renin activity (PRA), than those with a low PRA. [32] The antihypertensive action mainly depends on the blockade of the beta$_1$-AR, and the decreasement in the cardiac output is the major hemodynamic cause of the chronic reduction in blood pressure. Thus, the additional blockade of the beta$_2$-AR with propranolol does not provide a significant additional therapeutic benefit in coronary heart diseases (CHD), heart failures and lowering blood pressures. The initial negative cardiac depression may induce a reflex vasoconstriction to prevent blood pressure fall, but peripheral resistances returns quickly to baseline values and blood pressure falls. [1] The stimulation of the alpha-AR with NR increases the peripheral vasoconstriction, but in contrast the NR also stimulates the beta$_2$-AR and causes vasodilatation. Rascher and associates documented an increase in the vascular resistance, due to the beta$_2$-AR blockade, for concentrations of 0.01 μg/ml of propranolol. At concentrations of 10μg/ml of propranolol, vasodilatation occurred. The study was conducted in isolated perfused hindlimbs of rats. [34]

In 10 healthy males, orthostatic stress was simulated by the technique of the lower body negative pressure (LBNP). The forearm vascular resistance was measured in the control state and during LBNP at -10 and -40 mm Hg, with and without the administration of propranolol (0.1 mg/kg IV). Propranolol significantly reduced the reflex increase in the forearm vascular resistance, during LBNP at -40 mm Hg. This effect is probably a consequence of the propranolol induced decrease, in the activity of cardiac ventricular baroreceptors. [35]

In patients with cirrhosis and large- or medium sized varices, propranolol significantly reduces risk of the first variceal bleeding. In portal hypertension, a decrease in hepatic venous pressure gradient (HVPG) < 12 mm Hg essentially eliminates the risk of hemorrhage, and improves survival chances. [36] Increased levels of NR and ADR in cirrhosis stimulate the beta$_2$-AR, which contributes to further increases in the portal pressure. The beta$_2$-AR blockade with propranolol leads to unopposed alpha-AR vasoconstriction in the mesenteric arterioles. This results with an increase in the splanchnic and hepatic arterial resistance, with a simultaneous fall in the portal blood flow and the hepatic portal resistance. The propranolol reduction in the cardiac output further decreases the portal pressure. [37, 38]

The release of renin is mediated mainly by the beta$_1$-AR. However, the beta$_2$-AR are also involved, only to a lesser extent. [39] Propranolol inhibits the renin and aldosterone secretion, which both contribute to lowering the blood pressure. [32] Propranolol impairs the renal perfusion, due to a decrease in the cardiac output and the renal perfusion pressure. The alpha$_1$-AR vasoconstriction is stimulated and the renal vascular resistance (RVR) is increased, because of the propranolol mediated non-selective beta-AR blockade. The RVR contributes to a decrease in the renal perfusion as well. In addition, the reduced glomerular filtration rate (GFR) is documented in the chronic treatment with propranolol, also as a consequence of the decreased cardiac output. [40]

After propranolol treatments, an increased platelet aggregability was restored in patients with angina and abnormal exercise tolerance. [41] Long-term administration of propranolol led to a reduction of the ADP-induced platelet aggregation, thus it may prevent the venous thrombotic process. [42]

Propranolol rapidly ameliorates many of the symptoms of thyrotoxicosis, including palpitations, tachycardia, tremulousness and heat intolerance. Mechanisms, however, remain unclear. Propranolol inhibits the sympathetic activity. However, the thyrotoxicosis sympathetic nervous system and the adrenal medulla are normally active, with normal or even low circulating concentrations and urinary excretion of catecholamines. Also, there is no alteration in the catecholamine sensitivity during the beta-blockade, and the increase in the beta-AR is controversial. [43] Propranolol inhibits the 5'-monodeiodinase (type I and type II) that converts T4 to T3. [44] Its additional effect, via the inhibition of monodeiodinase type I, may cause T4 to be shunted through monodeiodinase type III and result in the production of the inactive reverse triiodothyronine (rT3). [45] Due to a high lipophilicity, propranolol becomes sufficiently concentrated in tissues to inhibit a 5'-monodeiodinase activity, but this effect occurs relatively slow, from 7-10 days. [46] In the euthyroid volunteers, who used propranolol 160 mg/day (or higher), it sustained as light rise in T4 and rT3, while T3 for a dose of 160 mg/day remained stable. It significantly fell for the dose of 240 mg/day. [47] In thyrotoxic patients, propranolol in doses of 160 mg/day or higher decreased the T3 concentrations for 30%. [48] Tagami and associates compared patients suffering from the Graves' disease, receiving methimazole either alone or in a combination with propranolol (doses of 30 or 60 mg/day). After 4 weeks of treatment, the group receiving the combination was documented to have a lower heart rate and improvements in various physical and psychical functions. [49]

Propranolol blocks the central and peripheral beta$_2$-AR, and the central serotonin (5-HT) receptors, which are all involved in the central nervous systems adverse reactions. [50] The results of the randomized controlled trial (RCT) demonstrated, that the S (-) enantiomer of propranolol decreases the production of nocturnal melatonin via a specific inhibition of the beta$_1$-AR, and consequently might be cause of sleep disturbances. [51]

The mechanisms of propranolol anti-migraine effects have not been established. One hypothesis is due to the inhibition of the cerebral vasospasm and the arteriolar spasm. [52] The propranolol effect on declarative memory is not clear. Maheu and associates have reported impaired declarative memory after propranolol treatments. [53] Van Stegeren and associates have reported that it affects only women, while Weymar and associates have not found any effects of propranolol, using male-only samples. [54, 55] In addition, Lonergan and associates reported the central inhibitory effect on the synthesis of proteins, which are necessary to consolidate new learning to the long-term memory storage after propranolol treatments. [56]

In vitro studies demonstrated propranolol antioxidant effects. It inhibits lipid peroxidation and glutathione depletion. [57] One mechanism, regarding a hypothesis, is due to the inhibition of xanthine oxidase, however it is controversial. [58, 59] The major metabolite of propranolol, 4-hydroxy-propranolol (4HOP), demonstrated a concentration-dependent inhibition of lipid peroxidation, in isolated hepatic microsomal membranes. It is 4- to 8- fold more potent than vitamin E, and >100-fold more active than propranolol. [60] However, in most of the studies, the used concentrations were much higher (20-200 μM) than peak plasma concentrations, that appear in clinical treatments with propranolol (~1 μM). [58-61]. The usage of propranolol may not be sufficient to provide antioxidant activities, correspondingly.

Due to a beta$_2$-AR blockade, by unmasking the parasympathetic and other bronchoconstrictor factors, propranolol may induce bronchospasm. [1] It also promotes the degranulation of mast cells and depresses the central responsiveness to carbon dioxide (CO_2). [62] Propranolol was given to 11 patients with a chronic obstructive pulmonary disease. In 2 patients, 10 mg IV of propranolol caused a reduction in the forced expiry volume (FEV_1), followed with dyspnea, cough and dizziness. In 5 other patients, 40 mg q.i.d of propranolol caused dyspnea. [63] It potentiates the bronchospasm, induced by histamine and acetylcholine. [64] Propranolol also reduced the FEV_1 by 2.4%, in patients with mild-to-moderate asthma. [65]

Propranolol is reducing the basal metabolic rate and thermogenesis by the beta-AR blockade. It causes weight gaining (~2-5 kg/year), that can be a predisposition to obesity. [66, 67] Propranolol reduces the lipoprotein lipase activity in the skeletal muscles. This explains the pronounced increase of the serum triglyceride (TG) concentration during propranolol treatments, despite lower free fatty acids and a higher lipoprotein lipase activity in the adipose tissue. [68] In scientific literature, a decrease in high density lipoprotein cholesterol concentrations has been reported, that also showed an increase in low density lipoprotein cholesterol (LDL-C) and very low density lipoprotein cholesterol (VLDL-C) concentrations. [69-70] In the Colombian population, subjects with Gln27Glu polymorphism (particularly homozygous for Gln27) for the ADRB2 gene that is encoding the $beta_2$-AR, show a significant reduction in HDL-C and an increase in TG after propranolol treatments. [71]

The beta-AR blockade leads to a decreased glucagon secretion, glycogenolysis and gluconeogenesis, while the alpha-AR stimulation inhibits the insulin secretion, glucagon secretion and enhances liver glycogenolysis. [72] The propranolol treatment decreased the insulin sensitivity index by 34%, and increased the HbA1c and glucose concentrations. [68] It also decreases the first phase of the insulin secretion, possibly due to an impairment of the beta2-AR-mediated insulin release. [68, 73]

Propranolol diminished the hyperglycemic response to ADR in healthy young volunteers, and abolished the ADR induced increase in lactate and pyruvate, ant the decrease in blood phosphorus and K^+. [74]

The stimulation of $beta_2$-AR induces the relaxation of the uterine muscle. In 73 nulliparous, pregnant women were exposed to 20 mg of oral propranolol, which increased the uterine activity to shorten the labor duration and reduced the frequency of the cesarean section. [75] The results of the RCT concluded that propranolol may shorten the induction duration and labor, and reduce the amount of necessary oxytocin. [76]

Propranolol lowers the intraocular pressure, due to the $beta_2$-AR blockade, by reducing the production of aqueous humor. [77, 78]

The $beta_2$-AR stimulation by ADR is reducing the potassium (K^+) plasma levels, by enhancing the K^+ entry in the skeletal muscle, and it can consequently induce tremor. Therefore, the $beta_2$-AR blockade with propranolol is a potential mechanism for reducing essential tremor. [79, 80]

The $beta_2$-AR blockade caused by propranolol, through the same mechanism as stated above, is also responsible for hyperkalemia in end-stage renal disease patients. [81]

Functional $beta_2$-ARs are documented in osteoblasts and osteoclasts, and sympathetic nerve fibers in bone tissue as well. [82, 83] Recent evidence suggests that the $beta_2$-AR activation in osteoblasts suppresses the osteogenic activity. [84] In the experiment where rats were used, the results presented a sympathetic system inactivation, which resulted in a significant decrease in the osteoclast number and activity. [85] *In vitro* propranolol caused a 1.5-fold increase in the proliferation of human osteoblastic cells, while in mice it increased their bone formation and bone mass. [86, 87] In postmenopausal woman, the usage of propranolol (160mg/day) reduced the serum osteocalcin (marker of bone turnover) by almost 20% in the first 2 weeks of treatment, and this effect increased over time. [88] These findings suggest that the nervous system is involved in the bone metabolism. Schlienger and associates have reported in their case control study, that the current use of beta-blockers is associated with a reduced risk of fractures. When taken alone, they reduce the relative risk for 23%, while in combination with thiazide diuretics, they reduce it by 29%. [89] The tumor necrosis factor alpha (TNF-alpha) increases the expression of the beta$_2$-AR in osteoblasts, and the expression of the receptor activator of the nuclear factor-kappaB ligand (RANKL), which is an essential osteoclastogenic factor. Due to the blockade of the beta$_2$-AR, propranolol blocked *in vitro* the suppression of osteogenic differentiation and stimulation of RANKL expression by TNF-alpha. [90]

Maisel and associates documented an interesting finding. After propranolol treatments, the impaired sympathetic activity (in healthy adult volunteers) markedly reduced the natural killer (NK) cells activity, concluding that propranolol can modulate the parameters of human immunity. [91]

Wanderley and associates documented *in vitro* using rat testicular interstitial cells, that propranolol increases the phosphorylation of histone by protein kinase C, and activates and stimulates the testosterone secretion by Leydig cells. The mechanism is possible by increasing the concentration of a chemical mediator, interacting with the regulatory domain of the protein kinase C. The relevance of this finding has yet to be determined, considering the fact that the study is made *in vitro*. [92] Another study demonstrated increased levels of testosterone in human models. Propranolol was given in 80 mg doses, two times a day (b.i.d.), for 6 weeks to 8 healthy young male medical students. The blood samples were taken overnight. Propranolol significantly reduced the plasma levels of the prolactin and luteinising hormone (LH), and it increased the plasma levels of testosterone. It is known that prolactin causes a renal salt and water retention, enhances the vasoconstrictor response to NR and that it increases the cellular levels of Na^+. These findings could at least partly be due to a direct central effect of propranolol. [93]

Nattel and associates reported the delayed onset and potentially long duration of the beta-AR hypersensitivity, after abrupt cessation of chronic treatments (3 months or longer) with propranolol, for essential hypertension in 9 studied patients. [94] On the other hand, in the normal subjects phenomenon of the beta-AR, hypersensitivity did not occur. Healthy 12 subjects received propranolol orally in doses of 120mg a day (for one week), and 6 days after abrupt cessation, measurements of the heart rate and blood pressure have been taken. There was no measurable increase in any of the parameters. [95] The propranolol withdrawal phenomenon is most likely due to the beta-AR hypersensitivity, which is the consequence of the increase in the beta-AR density during chronic treatments with propranolol. [96]

The beta$_1$-AR and beta$_2$-AR are expressed in the human infantile haemangioma (IH) endothelial cells. [97] Propranolol is used for treatments of IH, and several mechanisms are proposed. It decreases the expression of the hypoxia-inducible factor 1alpha (HIF-1alpha) and proangiogenic factors. Oxygen deficiency leads to an increase of the intracellular concentration of HIF-1alphain in its active form.

HIF-1alpha is a transcriptional modulator of the vascular endothelial growth factor (VEGF) gene. VEGF, the basic fibroblast growth factor and Matrix Metalloproteinase 9, are all proangiogenic factors. [98-100] The beta-AR blockade leaves an unmasked alpha$_1$-AR. It results in a peripheral vasoconstriction, which is immediately visible as a change in color, associated with a palpable softening of the hemangioma. [100] *In vitro* studies, that investigate the propranolol effect of triggering apoptosis of capillary endothelial cells, are controversial. [97, 101] But the studies demonstrated a decrease of proliferation and migration of endothelial progenitor cells, to the site predisposed for IH formation. [97]

CD34+ endothelial progenitor cells of the micro vessels in proliferating IH, express the angiotensin-converting enzyme and the angiotensin II receptor-2. Itinteang and associates documented formations of blast like structures, which proliferate in the presence of angiotensin II cells. Thus, propranolol may promote involution of IH through decreased renin production. [102]

Pharmacokinetics of Propranolol

Absorption

Propranolol is a highly lipophilic drug and it is almost completely absorbed after oral administration. [103] Propranolol undergoes a high first-pass metabolism in the liver, and only ~25% of the oral dose reaches the systemic circulation. The peak plasma concentration (C_{max}) occurs about 1 to 4 hours (h) after an oral dose. [9] It seems that the first-pass metabolism of propranolol is faster for the R (+) enantiomer, therefore the S (-) enantiomer plasma concentrations are higher than those of the R (+) enantiomer. [104-106] In 9 healthy volunteers, who received 160 mg of racemic propranolol as a single dose and then once daily for 7 days, the area under the plasma concentration time curve (AUC) of R (+) enantiomer and S (-) enantiomer were higher after 7 days, than AUC after single dose. Attained propranolol plasma concentrations were quite variable among individuals. [107] An increase in concentrations during long-term treatments is probably due to the reduction in the hepatic blood flow. For doses from 40 to 160 mg, the relation between the dose and the AUC of plasma concentration is linear, but for doses higher than 160 mg the AUC will increase in a non-linear fashion. [1]

The racial differences occur in the propranolol absorption. The AUC was lower in African-Americans than in Caucasians. [108] The AUC in Caucasian cirrhotic patients is enhanced, because of the decline in the hepatic blood flow when compared to non-cirrhotic patients. In Malay cirrhotic patients the AUC is even higher than in Caucasians, because the plasma concentration of $alpha_1$ glycoprotein are lower. [109, 110] The oral bioavailability of the drug may be increased in children with Down's syndrome. [111]

The bioavailability of the long acting propranolol has been estimated to be 50-80% of the conventional tablet. [112]

The sublingual administration of propranolol increases the bioavailability by threefold, compared to the oral administration, probably as a consequence of the reduction of the first-pass effect, plus a faster drug absorption. The sublingual and oral propranolol showed a similar clinical efficacy. [113] The bioavailability of the intranasal administration is shown to be nearly complete (~100%). [114] Comparing the oral to the rectal administration of propranolol, in case of a rectal administration, a 2-fold higher plasma concentration was observed. [115]

Propranolol decreases the GFR and renal blood flow by lowering the cardiac output. It results with an increase in the sympathetic activity, and consequently increases the resistance in the systemic and renal blood vessels via the alpha-AR stimulation. [40] The C_{max}, after a single oral dose of 40 mg of propranolol in the chronic renal failure patients, was 2 to 3-fold higher compared to healthy subjects and patients undergoing a regular dialysis treatment. The data suggest a reduced hepatic extraction, in chronic renal failure patients. [116] Propranolol is not significantly dialyzable. [117] Thus, in patients with a renal impairment, caution must be exercised when starting treatment and selecting the initial dose. In the pediatric population in case of renal impairment, the usage of propranolol is not recommended. [9, 11]

In cirrhotic patients, receiving 160 mg of conventional and long-acting propranolol, the C_{max} was ~3 fold higher than observed in non-cirrhotic subjects, due to a reduced first pass effect and a slight decrease in the hepatic blood flow. Conventional propranolol demonstrated a higher C_{max} level than a long-acting.

In cirrhotic patients, $t_{1/2}$ is also increased. [118] Patients with liver cirrhosis, after the IV administration (1 mg) of propranolol, demonstrated a 1.8-fold increase in the AUC, a 1.8-fold increase in volume of the distribution (Vd) and a 3-fold increase in the elimination half-life ($t_{1/2}$), compared to healthy controls. After the oral administration (40 mg) of propranolol, a 6-fold increase in the AUC, a 4-fold in elimination $t_{1/2}$ and a 3-fold in bioavailability was documented. [119]

Protein-rich foods increase the bioavailability of propranolol by about 50%, with no change in time to reach peak concentration, plasma binding, the elimination $t_{1/2}$, or the amount of the unchanged drug in the urine. [12] For the IV dose of 0.1 mg/kg of propranolol, the high-protein meal increased the systemic clearance for 38%, while the oral dose of 80 mg of propranolol slightly decreased oral clearance, albeit not statistically significant. The oral bioavailability increased by 67%, because of a 34% increase in the hepatic blood flow. [120] Protein rich foods increased the bioavailability, but displayed many interindividual variations, from a decrease to a 2.5 fold increase. The protein-rich food effect is probably due to a reduced hepatic extraction of propranolol. [121]

Distribution

Approximately 90% of the circulating propranolol is bound to plasma proteins, whereas the S (-) enantiomer is preferentially bound to $alpha_1$ glycoprotein, and the R (+) enantiomer to albumin. [122, 123]

Significantly lower mean concentrations of $alpha_1$ glycoprotein in the fetus blood, compared to that in the maternal blood, resulted in much higher free fractions of propranolol in the fetal blood. [124] The plasma protein binding of propranolol is not influenced by the age and gender of the patients. [125] The propranolol volume of distribution (Vd) is approximately 4 l/kg, it crosses the blood-brain barrier and the placenta, and it is distributed into breast milk. Therefore, while taking propranolol, breast feeding is not recommended. Propranolol should also not be given during pregnancy, unless its use is essential. [11] In obese patients, the Vd of propranolol is increased by about 70%, because propranolol distributes in excessive body weight, due to high lipophilicity. Consequently, the elimination $t_{1/2}$ increased also for 70%.

However, the oral absorption rate is the same for both groups, and the bioavailability is higher in obese patients (35% versus 27%), but the difference is not significant. Thus, the mean concentration in steady state will be the same in obese as in non-obese patients. [126] The trans-epithelial permeability (absorption and elimination) of propranolol is not affected by the P-glycoprotein (P-gp), but *in vitro* propranolol stimulated the P-gp expression in gut epithelial cells. [127]

Metabolism

Propranolol is metabolized through three primary routes:

- Propranolol naphthalene ring-hydroxylations (on the 4th, 5th, 7thposition) are contributing to 42% of the total metabolism of propranolol, and the main metabolite is 4HOPwhich also is an active metabolite. Because of the active 4HOP metabolite, 2 h after dosing, propranolol appears more potent that its plasma levels would suggest. Aromatic hydroxylation of propranolol is catalyzed mainly by polymorphic CYP2D6. [128-130]
- N-dealkylation, followed by further side-chain oxidation, is contributing to 41% of the total metabolism of propranolol. The main metabolite is the naphthoxylactic acid, catalyzed mainly by CYP1A2. [128-130]
- Direct glucuronidation is contributing to the remaining metabolism, with propranolol glucuronide as a metabolite. The glucuronic acid and sulfate conjugates of 4HOP are other main metabolites of propranolol. [11, 130]

In addition, CYP2C19 is also involved in the propranolol metabolism, just to a lesser extent. [11] Oral clearance and elimination $t_{1/2}$ of propranolol were not different, between the CYP2D6 extensive metabolizer and the poor metabolizer. Compared with poor metabolizers, the only difference was in the partial metabolic clearances of propranolol, being higher regarding the 4HOP concentrations and being lower regarding the naphthyloxylactic acid in extensive metabolizers. According to authors, CYP2D6 mediates approximately 65% and 70% of the propranolol S (-) enantiomer and the R (+) enantiomer 4-hydroxylation, respectively. [131]

In the pediatric population, the 4HOP was quantified, and its plasma exposure accounted for less than 7% of the parent drug exposure. [11]

Elimination

The plasma $t_{1/2}$ of propranolol ranges from 3 to 6 h. [129] The chronic use of propranolol decreases the hepatic blood flow and increases the elimination $t_{1/2}$. [122] Long acting propranolol has a prolonged t1/2 (8 to 11h), due to a slower absorption from the gut. [132] If racial differences are considered, the clearance was higher in black than in white subjects. [108]

Less than 1% of propranolol is excreted as an unchanged drug in the urine. [11] In 33 young healthy men, after a single 80 mg oral dose of propranolol, there was a positive correlation between the testosterone levels and the propranolol clearances. It happened through the alpha-naphthoxylactic acid and propranolol glucuronide, as well as the total clearance, but not through the aromatic ring hydroxylation. In addition, the propranolol clearance increased through the alpha-naphthoxylactic acid in 9 of 11 men, after administration of testosterone cypionate. Women showed no change in the propranolol clearance. Therefore, testosterone levels may be clinically relevant for propranolol therapies. [133]

In geriatric patients, the share of a fat tissue (relative to water) is increased, while lipophilic drugs, such as propranolol, accumulate more. In addition, kidneys are less able to excrete drugs into the urine and the liver is less able to metabolize drugs, which also contributes to enhanced propranolol accumulation. [134] Propranolol was given q.i.d. in single oral doses of 40 mg, single IV infusions of 0.15 mg/kg, and nine oral doses of 40 mg to healthy old and young subjects.

Comparing elderly subjects with younger subjects, they had higher plasma concentrations, longer elimination $t_{1/2}$ after the IV dose, and a greater bioavailability after the oral and IV dose. The differences in pharmacokinetics are existent because of the slower distribution of propranolol to tissues, and the diminished clearance in elderly subjects. [135] Inverse correlation was found between elderly patients and the partial metabolic clearances to the 4HOP and to naphthoxylactic acid, but no correlation with conjugation to propranolol glucuronide. Thus, the oxidation capacity probably declines with age, but the conjugation capacity remains unaltered. [136]

In the pediatric population, the mean oral clearance was 2.71 l/h/kg in infants aged 65-120 days, and 3.27 l/h/kg in infants aged 181- 240 days. [11]

Oral versus parenteral doses exist in a ~ 40:1 ratio, due to a high first-pass metabolism in the liver. [122] For the IV administration of propranolol, starting doses are 1-3 mg and the hepatic extraction is so efficient that the propranolol clearance is dependent on the liver blood flow. [103] After the IV administration of 20 mg of propranolol in 6 young healthy volunteers, the mean distribution $t_{1/2}$ was~17.4 minutes (min) and elimination $t_{1/2}$~5.3 h. [137] After a single IV dose (8 mg) of propranolol to obese and non-obese patients, the elimination $t_{1/2}$ was similar. [138]

Pharmacokinetic Interactions

There are 2 major mechanisms that are responsible for cytochrome P450–mediated drug interactions. The conversion of a drug to inactive or active metabolites is a consequence of induction (increased synthesis or decreased degradation) of cytochrome P450 enzymes. Therefore, the induction decreases the plasma levels of drugs, and in the most cases its pharmacodynamic effects, with the exception of pro-drugs or drugs that have active metabolites.

The potent inhibition leads to either enzyme inactivation or mutual competition of substrates for a catalytic site. The decrease of the drug metabolism, prolongation of the elimination $t_{1/2}$, the enhancement of drug pharmacodynamic (or toxic) effects or lack of the pharmacodynamic effects (pro-drugs) follows, respectively. As stated before, propranolol is metabolized by CYP1A2, CYP2C19 and CYP2D6, thus its pharmacokinetics is strongly affected by cytochrome P450 inducers and inhibitors. The cytochrome P450 inducers of the propranolol metabolism are presented in Table 3. [139-144] The cytochrome P450 inhibitors of the propranolol metabolism are presented in Table 4. [144-149]

T4 can increase the propranolol metabolism, while antithyroid drugs and radio-iodine inhibit the propranolol metabolism and consequently increase the propranolol plasma concentration. [150] Propafenone significantly increased the C_{max}, time necessary to peak the plasma concentration (T_{max}), elimination $t_{1/2}$ and mean steady-state plasma concentrations

(C_{ss}) by 83%, 55%, 30% and 213%, respectively. [151] Propafenone is a potent inhibitor of CYP1A2, and according to some authors, it may cause a drug-drug interaction with drugs metabolized by CYP1A2. [152]

Hydralazin increased the C_{max} and the AUC of oral propranolol, due to an altering first-pass metabolism in the liver. [153] Lacidipine significantly increased the C_{max} (35%) and the AUC (26%) of oral propranolol, while the T_{max} and elimination $t_{1/2}$ were not affected. Thus, the pharmacokinetic interaction is evident, and cytochrome P450 enzymes are implicated. [154] Interestingly, the inhibitory effects of quinidine, verapamil, cimetidine and nicardipine on the propranolol metabolism were more stereoselective for the R (+) enantiomer, resulting in a significant increase in the R (+) enantiomer vs. the S (-) enantiomer AUC ratio in plasma. [106, 155-157] The plasma concentration of oral propranolol decreased after the administration of 2 doses of either cholestyramine or colestipol. The reason may be in the altered absorption phase of propranolol. [158] Propranolol was administrated IV, 1 mg/kg to rabbits. After the administration of oral activated charcoal, the elimination $t_{1/2}$ was reduced by 16.6%, the AUC by 14% and the systemic clearance increased by 17%, compared to the control group of animals. According to the authors, the activated charcoal probably interrupted the enterohepatic circulation. [159]

Table 3. Cytochrome P450 inducers of propranolol metabolism

CYP1A2 inducers	CYP2C19 inducers	CYP2D6 inducers	Interaction outcome
Rifampicin Phenobarbital	Rifampicin Phenytoin	Ethanol (induces CYP2D6 only in the brain but not in the liver)	May increase propranolol clearance

Table 4. Cytochrome P450 inhibitors of propranolol metabolism

CYP1A2 inhibitors	CYP2C19 inhibitors	CYP2D6 inhibitors	Interaction outcome
Chlorpromazine Cimetidine Fluvoxamine	Felbamate Fluconazole Fluoxetine Fluvoxamine MAO inhibitors Omeprazole Ticlopidine	Amiodarone Chlorpromazine Cimetidine Clomipramine Fluoxetine Haloperidol HIV protease inhibitors MAO inhibitors Mibefradil Norfluoxetine Paroxetine Quinidine Thioridazine	May increase propranolol plasma concentration and consequently exert toxic effects

Pharmacokinetic Interaction: The Effect of Propranolol on Other Drugs

The propranolol inhibited metabolism of intravenous lidocaine resulted in a ~25% increase in lidocaine concentrations and decreased clearance. Thus, it can increase the lidocaine toxicity (the neurological and cardiac adverse events). The CYP1A2 is the enzyme primarily responsible for the metabolic disposition of lidocaine, and propranolol is also a substrate for this enzyme, therefore the CYP1A2 may be implicated in the interaction mechanism. [160-162]

Oral propranolol also altered the pharmacokinetics of the calcium-channel blockers (CCB). It significantly decreased the C_{max} (38%) and the AUC (42%) of lacidipine, while in contrast it reduced the oral clearance by 51% and increased the oral bioavailability by 48% of diltiazem. [154, 163]

The thioridazine and chlorpromazine concentrations have been increased after the propranolol administration. [164, 165] Chlorpromazine is a substrate of CYP2D6 and CYP1A2, and thioridazine is a substrate of CYP2D6. [166, 167] Thus, there is a possibility that these enzymes may be implicated in the interaction mechanism, although this hypothesis has yet to be determined.

Oral propranolol caused a reduction in the clearance of diazepam which is biotransformed mainly by N-demethylation (CYP1A2). [168] It also reduced the clearance of bromazepam and the prolonged elimination $t_{1/2}$ (28 vs. 23 h). [169]

The propranolol treatment (120mg, twice daily, for 7.5 days) increased the C_{max} (75%) and the AUC (67%) of rizatriptan (5-$HT_{1B/1D}$ agonist). According to the authors, one possible mechanism is that propranolol, or its metabolite (N-desmethyl propranolol), competitively inhibits the enzyme monoamine oxidase A (MAO-A), which is involved in the metabolism of rizatriptan. [170] Peck and associates have shown that propranolol also increases the plasma concentrations of zolmitriptan, but authors state that there is no evidence that propranolol is a MAO inhibitor. [171]

Oral propranolol reduced, in a dose depended manner, the theophylline clearance between 30-52%, while cytochrome P-450 is implicated in the pharmacokinetic interaction. Propranolol also has an antagonistic effect on theophylline. [172, 173]

Pharmacodynamics Interactions

The interaction between amiodarone (a class III anti-arrhythmic drug) and propranolol is associated more with the electrophysiological (sinus bradycardia and sinus arrest) and/or haemodynamic toxicity, due to added pharmacological effects, than to changes in pharmacokinetics. Amiodarone induces the negative inotropic effect and it has a potentiating effect on the atrial-conduction time. [11, 174] Disopyramide (a class I anti-arrhythmic drug), in combination with propranolol, significantly decreased the heart rate, similarly as amiodarone, due to the potentiating effect on the atrial-conduction time and the induced negative inotropic effect. [9, 175] Propafenon has a negative inotropic effect and beta-AR blocking properties. Thus, there is a possibility that these properties can be added to propranolol. [11]

Digitalis slows atrioventricular conductions and decreases the heart rate, thus the concomitant usage with propranolol can induce hemodynamic interactions and increase the risk of bradycardia. [11, 176] The usage of propranolol with anesthetic drugs can depress the myocardial contractility and the vascular compensating response. [11]

Combined with propranolol, the dihydropyridine CCB may induce hypotension and/or heart failure, particularly in patients with increased cardiac sympathetic activity that compensates for a negative inotropic effect of CCB. [150]

The interactions between verapamil and propranolol may involve in negative chronotropic, inotropic, and dromotropic effects. The co-administration of propranolol with verapamil and diltiazem can lead to an exaggeration of these effects, particularly in patients with impaired ventricular function and/or SA or AV conduction abnormalities. [150, 177, 178] The co-administration of ACE-inhibitors, angiotensin II-receptors antagonists, diuretics, alpha-blockers or peripheral vasodilators with propranolol, can cause or increase hypotension. [150, 179-183] Propranolol may exacerbate the rebound hypertension, with the clonidine co-administration or in the case of the withdrawal of clonidine. The possible mechanism is related to the unopposed $alpha_1$-AR stimulation, which occurs as a consequence of a non-selective beta-AR blockade. In addition, clonidine stimulates the peripheral alpha-AR in higher doses. [183] Reserpine (a catecholamine-depleting drug), in combination with propranolol, can cause an excessive reduction of resting sympathetic nervous activity, which may result in hypotension, marked bradycardia, vertigo, syncope, or orthostatic hypotension. [184] A concomitant use of ADR and NR with propranolol may cause vasoconstriction, hypertension and bradycardia, due to an unopposed $alpha_1$-AR stimulation. [150, 185] The NSAID inhibits the synthesis of vasodilatory prostaglandins, that increase the renal blood flow and hence favors the excretion of water and sodium. Thus, the NSAID can blunt the antihypertensive effect of propranolol, although the changes in blood pressure are usually small (5-6 mmHg). [186] Propranolol, in combination with ergotamine, dihydroergotamine or related compounds, can produce manifestations of excessive vasoconstriction because of the blocking vasodilation pathways. [187] Propranolol, in combination with hypoglycaemic agents, may mask adrenalin-induced symptoms of hypoglycemia and prolong the hypoglycaemic response to insulin. [188] The concomitant use of corticosteroids and propranolol in IH can increase the risk of hypoglycaemia, due to an adrenal suppression by corticosteroids, which results in the loss of the counter regulatory cortisol response. [11]

The beta-AR agonists exert the reverse pharmacological effects of propranolol, mediated by the $beta_2$-AR. [189] Oral propranolol (40 mg) was effective in reversing the cardiovascular and metabolic effects of oral salbutamol (8 mg). [190]

Propranolol and ethanol demonstrated an additive depressor effect on night-time blood pressure. [191] As in combinations with CNS, depressants propranolol can also exacerbate orthostatic hypotension in the combination with ethanol. [139]

Conclusion

Since the propranolol discovery up until now, vast studies have documented its pharmacodynamics and pharmacokinetics. The pharmacodynamics of propranolol is based on a non-selective beta-AR blockade. The $beta_1$-AR blockade is responsible for most of the cardiovascular effects, and the additional $beta_2$-AR blockade does not provide any benefits in CHD, heart failure and lowering blood pressure. However, the $beta_2$-AR blockade is beneficial in the reduction of essential tremor, aqueous humor production, portal hypertension, treatment of IH and increase in the uterine activity to shorten the labor duration. The pharmacokinetics of propranolol is in a relation with high lipophilicity and a high first-pass hepatic metabolism. One of the reasons why propranolol is not used in cardiology as much as before, is because of non-selectivity. Propranolol is a substrate of CYP1A2, CYP2C19 and CYP2D6 cytochrome P450 enzymes. Some pharmacokinetic interactions of propranolol are more stereoselective for the R (+) enantiomer, but further studies are necessary to determine the clinical relevance of these findings. Besides pharmacokinetic interactions, there is also a vast number of pharmacodynamics interactions, mostly because of adjuvant synergistic or antagonistic effects. Nevertheless, propranolol still has its place in therapy, and it is unlikely to lose it. Recent discoveries in involution of IH with propranolol have put it into focus again, as angina pectoris treatments did 50 years ago.

References

[1] Lechat P. Clinical pharmacology of beta-blockers in cardiology: trial results and clinical applications. *Hot Topics in Cardiology*, 2008; 10:7-44.

[2] Granneman J. G. The putative beta4-adrenergic receptor is a novel state of the beta1-adrenergic receptor. *Am. J. Physiol. Endocrinol. Metab.,* 2001; 280(2):E199-202.

[3] Mccorry L. K. Physiology of the autonomic nervous system. *Am. J. Pharm. Educ.*, 2007; 71(4):78.

[4] Dzimiri N. Regulation of beta-adrenoceptor signaling in cardiac function and disease. *Pharmacol. Rev*., 1999; 51(3):465-501.

[5] Iaizzo P. A. Handbook of Cardiac Anatomy, Physiology, and Devices. Springer Science and Business Media; 2009.

[6] Hebb A. R., Godwin T. F., Gunn R. W. A new beta adrenergic blocking agent, propranolol, in the treatment of angina pectoris. *Can. Med. Assoc. J.*, 1968; 98(5): 246-51.

[7] Frishman W. H. Fifty years of beta-adrenergic blockade: a golden era in clinical medicine and molecular pharmacology. *Am. J. Med.,* 2008; 121 (11): 933-4.

[8] Baker J. G. The selectivity of beta-adrenoceptor antagonists at the human beta1, beta2 and beta3 adrenoceptors. *Br. J. Pharmacol.,* 2005; 144(3):317-22.

[9] Medicines and Healthcare Products Regulatory Agency [Internet]. London: Medicines and Healthcare Products Regulatory Agency; 2000 [updated 2011 Sep 1, cited 2014 Oct 2]; Medicines Information; Inderal; [About 7 screens]. Available from:http://www.mhra.gov.uk/home/groups/spcpil/documents/spcpil/con139538169281 1. pdf

[10] Roth B. L. The Serotonin Receptors, From Molecular Pharmacology to Human Therapeutics. Humana Press; 2006.

[11] European Medicines Agency [Internet]. London: European Medicines Agency; 2014 [cited 2014 Oct 1]. Hemangiol:EPAR-Product Information; [about 20 screens].

Available from: http:// www.ema.europa.eu/docs/en_GB/document_library/EPAR_-_Product_Information/human

[12] Barrett A. M., Cullum V. A. The biological properties of the optical isomers of propranolol and their effects on cardiac arrhythmias. *Br. J. Pharmacol.,* 1968; 34(1): 43-55.

[13] Stoschitzky K., Lindner W., Egginger G., et al. Racemic (R,S)-propranolol versus half-dosed optically pure (S)-propranolol in humans at steady state: Hemodynamic effects, plasma concentrations, and influence on thyroid hormone levels. *Clin. Pharmacol. Ther.,* 1992; 51 (4):445-53.

[14] Fagan T. C., Gourley L. A., Sawyer P. R., Lee J. T., Walle T., Gaffney T. E. Acute hypotensive effects of oral and intravenous propranolol: early alterations in peripheral resistance. *J. Clin. Hypertens.,* 1986; 2(1):21-9.

[15] Bodem G., Brammell H. L., Weil J. V., Chidsey C. A. Pharmacodynamic studies of beta adrenergic antagonism induced in man by propranolol and practolol. *J. Clin. Invest.*, 1973; 52(4):747-54.

[16] Clark M. A., Harvey R. A., Finkel R. et al. Pharmacology. Lippincott Williams & Wilkins; 2011.

[17] Black J. W., Duncan W. A., Shanks R. G. Comparison of some properties of pronethalol and propranolol. 1965. *Br. J. Pharmacol.,* 1997; 120(4 Suppl.):285-99.

[18] Shanks R. G. The Effect of Propranolol on the Cardiovascular Responses to Isoprenaline, Adrenaline and Noradrenaline in the Anesthetized Dog. *Br. J. Pharmacol. and Chemother.*, 1966; 26:322.

[19] Colin P., Ghaleh B., Hittinger L., et al. Differential effects of heart rate reduction and beta-blockade on left ventricular relaxation during exercise. *Am. J. Physiol. Heart Circ. Physiol.*, 2002; 282(2):H672-9.

[20] Jorgensen C. R., Wang K., Wang Y., Gobel F. L., Nelson R. R., Taylor H. Effect of propranolol on myocardial oxygen consumption and its hemodynamic correlates during upright exercise. *Circulation,* 1973; 48(6):1173-82.

[21] Pfizer Canada Inc. [Internet]. Quebec: Pfizer Canada Inc.; 2010 [updated 2012 Sep 14, cited 2014 Oct 4]; Product monograph; Inderal-LA; [About 7 screens]. Available from: http://www.pfizer.ca/en/ our_products/products/monograph/265

[22] Prystowsky E. N. The effects of slow channel blockers and beta blockers on atrioventricular nodal conduction. *J. Clin. Pharmacol.*, 1988; 28(1):6-21.

[23] Lucchesi B. R., Whitsitt L. S., Brown N. L. Propranolol in Experimentally Induced Cardiac Arrhythmias. *Can. J. Physiol. And Pharmacol.*, 1966; 44:543.

[24] Vila-petroff M., Pérez G. N., Alvarez B., Cingolani H. E., Mattiazzi A. Mechanism of negative lusitropic effect of alpha 1-adrenoceptor stimulation in cat papillary muscles. *Am. J. Physiol.*, 1996; 270(2 Pt 2):H701-9.

[25] Petroff M. V., Mundiña-weilenmann C., Vittone L., Chiappe de cingolani G., Mattiazzi A. Lusitropic effects of alpha- and beta-adrenergic stimulation in amphibian heart. *Mol. Cell Biochem.,* 1994; 141(2):87-95.

[26] Doggrell S. A. The membrane stabilizing and beta 1-adrenoceptor blocking activity of (+)- and (-)-propranolol on the rat left atria. *Gen. Pharmacol.*, 1990; 21(5):677-80.

[27] McDevitt D. G. The Assessment of Beta-Adrenoceptor Blocking Drugs in Man. *Br. J. Clin. Pharmac.*, 1977; 4:413-425.

[28] Iwai T., Tanonaka K., Kasahara S., Inoue R., Takeo S. Protective effect of propranolol on mitochondrial function in the ischaemic heart. *Br. J. Pharmacol.*, 2002; 136(3): 472-80.

[29] Sievert H., Frey G., Schräder R., et al. Influence of carvedilol and propranolol on coronary blood flow. *Eur. J. Clin. Pharmacol.*, 1990; 38 Suppl. 2:S122-4.

[30] Hiatt W. R., Stoll S., Nies A. S. Effect of beta-adrenergic blockers on the peripheral circulation in patients with peripheral vascular disease. *Circulation,* 1985; 72(6): 1226-31.

[31] Paravastu S. C., Mendonca D. A., Da silva A. Beta blockers for peripheral arterial disease. *Cochrane Database Syst. Rev.,* 2013; 9:CD005508.

[32] Bühler F. R., Laragh J. H., Baer L., Vaughan E. D., Brunner H. R. Propranolol inhibition of renin secretion. A specific approach to diagnosis and treatment of renin-dependent hypertensive diseases. *N. Engl. J. Med.*, 1972; 287(24):1209-14.

[33] Struyker-boudier H. A., Smits J. F. Antihypertensive action of beta-adrenoceptor blocking drugs. The role of intrarenal mechanisms. *Am. J. Hypertens.*, 1989; 2(11 Pt 2):237S-240S.

[34] Rascher W., Mann J. F., Schömig A., Dietz R., Lüth J. B. Effects of beta-adrenergic blocking agents on peripheral vascular resistance. *Klin. Wochenschr.*, 1978; 56 Suppl. 1:87-90.

[35] Ferguson D. W., Thames M. D., Mark A. L. Effects of propranolol on reflex vascular responses to orthostatic stress in humans. Role of ventricular baroreceptors. *Circulation,* 1983; 67(4):802-7.

[36] Garcia-tsao G., Sanyal A. J., Grace N. D., Carey W. Prevention and management of gastroesophageal varices and variceal hemorrhage in cirrhosis. *Hepatology,* 2007; 46(3):922-38.

[37] Toubia N., Sanyal A. J. Portal hypertension and variceal hemorrhage. *Med. Clin. North Am.*, 2008; 92(3):551-74, viii.

[38] Bihari D., Westaby D., Gimson A., Crossley I., Harry J., Williams R. Reductions in portal pressure by selective beta 2-adrenoceptor blockade in patients with cirrhosis and portal hypertension. *Br. J. Clin. Pharmacol.*, 1984; 17(6):753-7.

[39] Gaál K., Mózes T., Rohla M. The role of beta receptors in the regulation of renin release. *Acta Physiol. Acad. Sci. Hung.,* 1979; 54(3):295-302.

[40] Epstein M., Oster J. R. Beta blockers and renal function: a reappraisal. *J. Clin. Hypertens.*, 1985; 1(1):85-99.

[41] Frishman W. H., Weksler B., Christodoulou J. P., Smithen C., Killip T. Reversal of abnormal platelet aggregability and change in exercise tolerance in patients with angina pectoris following oral propranolol. *Circulation,* 1974; 50(5):887-96.

[42] Gruszecki M., Ró³kowski R., Pawlak R., Buczko W. Propranolol prevents the development of venous thrombosis in rats by a platelet-dependent mechanism. *Pol. J. Pharmacol.*, 2001; 53(1):5-10.

[43] Geffner D. L., Hershman J. M. Beta-adrenergic blockade for the treatment of hyperthyroidism. *Am. J. Med.,* 1992; 93(1):61-8.

[44] Wiersinga W. M. Propranolol and thyroid hormone metabolism. *Thyroid,* 1991; 1(3):273-7.

[45] Kallner G., Ljunggren J. G., Tryselius M. The effect of propranolol on serum levels of T4, T3 and reverse-T3 in hyperthyroidism. *Acta Med. Scand.*, 1978; 204(1-2):35-7.

[46] Perrild H., Hansen J. M., Skovsted L., Christensen L. K. Different effects of propranolol, alprenolol, sotalol, atenolol and metoprolol on serum T3 and serum rT3 in hyperthyroidism. *Clin. Endocrinol. (Oxf.),* 1983; 18(2):139-42.

[47] Wilkins M. R., Franklyn J. A., Woods K. L., Kendall M. J. Effect of propranolol on thyroid homeostasis of healthy volunteers. *Postgrad. Med. J.*, 1985; 61(715):391-4.

[48] Franklyn J. A., Wilkins M. R., Wilkinson R., Ramsden D. B., Sheppard M. C. The effect of propranolol on circulating thyroid hormone measurements in thyrotoxic and euthyroid subjects. *Acta Endocrinol.,* 1985; 108(3):351-5.

[49] Tagami T., Yambe Y., Tanaka T., et al. Short-term effects of β-adrenergic antagonists and methimazole in new-onset thyrotoxicosis caused by Graves' disease. *Intern. Med.*, 2012; 51(17):2285-90.

[50] Yamada, Y., Shibuya, F., Hamada, J. et al. Prediction of sleep disorders induced by beta-adrenergic receptor blocking agents based on receptor occupancy. *J. Pharmacokinet. Biopharm.*, 1995; 23: 131–145.

[51] Stoschitzky K., Sakotnik A., Lercher P., et al. Influence of beta-blockers on melatonin release. *Eur. J. Clin. Pharmacol.*, 1999; 55(2):111-5.

[52] Ouellette R., Joyce J. Pharmacology for Nurse Anesthesiology. Jones and Bartlett Publishers; 2010.

[53] Maheu F. S., Joober R., Beaulieu S., Lupien S. J. Differential effects of adrenergic and corticosteroid hormonal systems on human short- and long-term declarative memory for emotionally arousing material. *Behav. Neurosci.*, 2004; 118(2):420-8.

[54] Van Stegeren A. H., Goekoop R., Everaerd W., et al. Noradrenaline mediates amygdala activation in men and women during encoding of emotional material. *Neuroimage,* 2005; 24:898–909.

[55] Weymar M., Low A., Modess C., et al. Propranolol selectively blocks the enhanced parietal old/new effect during long-term recollection of unpleasant pictures: a high density ERP study. *Neuroimage,* 2010; 49:2800–6.

[56] Lonergan M. H., Olivera-figueroa L. A., Pitman R. K., Brunet A. Propranolol's effects on the consolidation and reconsolidation of long-term emotional memory in healthy participants: a meta-analysis. *J. Psychiatry Neurosci.*, 2013; 38(4):222-31.

[57] Denisov E. T., Afanas'ev I. B. Oxidation and Antioxidants in Organic Chemistry and Biology. CRC Press; 2005.

[58] Janero D. R., Lopez R., Pittman J., Burghardt B. Propranolol as xanthine oxidase inhibitor: implications for antioxidant activity. *Life Sci.,* 1989; 44(21):1579-88.

[59] Aruoma O. I., Smith C., Cecchini R., Evans P. J., Halliwell B. Free radical scavenging and inhibition of lipid peroxidation by beta-blockers and by agents that interfere with calcium metabolism. A physiologically-significant process? *Biochem. Pharmacol.*, 1991; 42(4):735-43.

[60] Mak I. T., Weglicki W. B. Potent antioxidant properties of 4-hydroxyl-propranolol. *J. Pharmacol. Exp. Ther.*, 2004; 308(1):85-90.

[61] Zal F., Taheri R., Khademi F., Keshavarz E., Rajabi S., Mostafavi-pour Z. The combined effect of furosemide and propranolol on GSH homeostasis in ACHN renal cells. *Toxicol. Mech. Methods,* 2014; 24(6): 412-6.

[62] Trembath P. W., Taylor E. A., Varley J., Turner P. Effect of propranolol on the ventilatory response to hypercapnia in man. *Clin. Sci.,* 1979; 57(5): 465-8.

[63] Tivenius L., Nyberg G. Effect of Alprenolol and Propranolol on ventilatory function. A comparative Study in Patients With Chronic Obstructive Lung Disease. *Pharmacologia Clinica*, 1969; 2:51.

[64] Dixon E. J., Wilsoncroft P., Robertson D. N., Page C. P. The effect of Paf antagonists on bronchial hyperresponsiveness induced by Paf, propranolol or indomethacin. *Br. J. Pharmacol.*, 1989; 97(3):717-22.

[65] Short P. M., Williamson P. A., Anderson W. J., Lipworth B. J. Randomized placebo-controlled trial to evaluate chronic dosing effects of propranolol in asthma. *Am. J. Respir. Crit. Care Med.,* 2013; 187 (12): 1308-14.

[66] Rössner S., Taylor C. L., Byington R. P., Furberg C. D. Long term propranolol treatment and changes in body weight after myocardial infarction. *BMJ*, 1990; 300(6729):902-3.

[67] Astrup A. V. [Obesity and diabetes as side-effects of beta-blockers]. *Ugeskr. Laeg.*, 1990; 152(40):2905-8.

[68] Lithell H., Pollare T., Vessby B. Metabolic effects of pindolol and propranolol in a double-blind cross-over study in hypertensive patients. *Blood Press.,* 1992; 1(2):92-101.

[69] Fogari R., Zoppi A., Tettamanti F., et al. Beta-blocker effects on plasma lipids in antihypertensive therapy: importance of the duration of treatment and the lipid status before treatment. *J. Cardiovasc. Pharmacol.*, 1990; 16 Suppl. 5:S76-80.

[70] Samuel P., Chin B., Schoenfeld B. H., Schaefer E. J., Gonasun L. M. Comparison of the effect of pindolol vs propranolol on the lipid profile in patients treated for hypertension. *Br. J. Clin. Pharmacol.*, 1987; 24 Suppl. 1:63S-64S.

[71] Isaza C., Henao J., Ramirez E., Cuesta F., Cacabelos R. Polymorphic variants of the beta2-adrenergic receptor (ADRB2) gene and ADRB2-related propanolol-induced dyslipidemia in the Colombian population. *Methods Find Exp. Clin. Pharmacol.*, 2005; 27(4):237-44.

[72] Mills G. A., Horn J. R. Beta-blockers and glucose control. *Drug Intell. Clin. Pharm.*, 1985; 19(4):246-51.

[73] Kaneto A., Miki E., Kosaka K. Effect of beta and beta2 adrenoreceptor stimulants infused intrapancreatically on glucagon and insulin secretion. *Endocrinology,* 1975; 97(5):1166-73.

[74] Massara F., Camanni F., Molinatti G. Effect of propranolol on some adrenaline- and insulin-induced metabolic changes in man. *Acta Diabetol. Lat.,* 1975; 12(1):41-51.

[75] Direkvand-Moghadam A., Jaafarpour M., Khani A., Taheri S., Delpisheh A. The effect of oral propranolol plus oxytocin versus oxytocin only on the process and outcome of labor: A double-blind randomized trial. *Iran J. Nurs. Midwifery Res.,* 2014; 19(5): 491-5.

[76] Kashanian M., Fekrat M., Zarrin Z., Ansari N. S. A comparison between the effect of oxytocin only and oxytocin plus propranolol on the labor (a double blind randomized trial). *J. Obstet. Gynaecol. Res.,* 2008; 34(3): 354-8.

[77] Nathanson J. A. Adrenergic regulation of intraocular pressure: identification of beta 2-adrenergic-stimulated adenylate cyclase in ciliary process epithelium. *Proc. Natl. Acad. Sci. USA*, 1980; 77(12):7420-4.

[78] Wygnanski-Jaffe T., Spierer A., Melamed S., Ben-zion I. The effect of oral propranolol on intraocular pressure in infants with Sturge-Weber syndrome glaucoma. *Eur. J. Ophthalmol.*, 2015; 25(2).

[79] Calzetti S., Findley L. J., Perucca E., Richens A. The response of essential tremor to propranolol: evaluation of clinical variables governing its efficacy on prolonged administration. *J. Neurol. Neurosurg. Psychiatr.*, 1983; 46(5):393-8.

[80] Tesfamariam B., Waldron T., Seymour A. A. Quantitation of tremor in response to beta-adrenergic receptor stimulation in primates: relationship with hypokalemia. *J. Pharmacol. Toxicol. Methods*, 1998; 40(4):201-5.

[81] Allon M. Hyperkalemia in end-stage renal disease: mechanisms and management. *J. Am. Soc. Nephrol.*, 1995; 6(4):1134-42.

[82] Togari A., Arai M., Mizutani S., Koshihara Y., Nagatsu T. Expression of mRNAs for neuropeptide receptors and beta-adrenergic receptors in human osteoblasts and human osteogenic sarcoma cells. *Neurosci. Lett.,* 1997; 233:125-128.

[83] Togari A. Adrenergic regulation of bone metabolism: possible involvement of sympathetic innervation of osteoblastic and osteoclastic cells. *Microsc. Res. Tech.,* 2002; 58:77-84.

[84] Fu L., Patel M. S., Bradley A., Wagner E. F., Karsenty G. The molecular clock mediates leptin-regulated bone formation. *Cell,* 2005; 122(5): 803-15.

[85] Cherruau M., Morvan F. O., Schirar A., Saffar J. L. Chemical sympathectomy-induced changes in TH-, VIP-, and CGRP-immunoreactive fibers in the rat mandible periosteum: influence on bone resorption. *J. Cell Physiol.*, 2003; 194:341-348.

[86] Teong B., Kuo S. M., Chen C. H., Chen Y. K., Cheng Z. J., Huang H. H. Characterization and human osteoblastic proliferation- and differentiation-stimulatory effects of phosphatidylcholine liposomes-encapsulated propranolol hydrochloride. *Biomed. Mater. Eng.,* 2014; 24(5): 1875-87.

[87] Takeda S., Elefteriou F., Levasseur R. et al. Leptin regulates bone formation via the sympathetic nervous system. *Cell,* 2002; 111:305-317.

[88] Reid I. R., Lucas J., Wattie D., et al. Effects of a beta-blocker on bone turnover in normal postmenopausal women: a randomized controlled trial. *J. Clin. Endocrinol. Metab.*, 2005; 90(9):5212-6.

[89] Schlienger R. G., Kraenzlin M. E., Jick S. S., Meier C. R. Use of beta-blockers and risk of fractures. *JAMA*, 2004; 292(11):1326-32.

[90] Baek K., Lee H. L., Hwang H. R., Park H. J., Kwon A., Qadir A. S., Baek J. H. TNFalpha Increases the Expression of beta2 Adrenergic Receptors in Osteoblasts. *Int. J. Oral. Biol.*, 2011; 36(4):173-178.

[91] Maisel A. S., Murray D., Lotz M., Rearden A., Irwin M., Michel M. C. Propranolol treatment affects parameters of human immunity. *Immunopharmacology*, 1991; 22(3):157-64.

[92] Wanderley M. I., Udrisar D. P., Martins M. C., Antunes-rodrigues J. Propranolol stimulates histone phosphorylation by a putative PK-C in partially purified homogenate of rat testicular interstitial cells. A possible mechanism for increased testosterone secretion by propranolol. *Horm. Metab. Res.,* 2000; 32(7):259-64.

[93] Dart A. M., Lewis M. J., Groom G. V., Meek E. M., Henderson A. H. The effect of chronic propranolol treatment on overnight plasma levels of anterior pituitary and related hormones. *Br. J. Clin. Pharmacol.,* 1981; 12(6):849-53.

[94] Nattel S., Rangno R. E., Van loon G. Mechanism of propranolol withdrawal phenomena. *Circulation,* 1979; 59(6):1158-64.

[95] Kiyingi K. S., Shaw J. The phenomenon of beta-adrenergic hypersensitivity following propranolol withdrawal studied in normal subjects. *Eur. J. Clin. Pharmacol.*, 1984; 27(4):423-8.

[96] Aarons R. D., Nies A. S., Gal J., Hegstrand L. R., Molinoff P. B. Elevation of beta-adrenergic receptor density in human lymphocytes after propranolol administration. *J. Clin. Invest.*, 1980; 65(5):949-57.

[97] Stiles J., Amaya C., Pham R., et al. Propranolol treatment of infantile hemangioma endothelial cells: A molecular analysis. *Exp. Ther. Med.,* 2012; 4(4):594-604.

[98] Hassan B. A., Shreef K. S. Propranolol in treatment of huge and complicated infantile hemangiomas in egyptian children. *Dermatol. Res. Pract.*, 2014; 2014:541810.

[99] Storch C. H., Hoeger P. H. Propranolol for infantile haemangiomas: insights into the molecular mechanisms of action. *Br. J. Dermatol.,* 2010; 163(2):269-74.

[100] Léauté-Labrèze C., Dumas de la Roque E., Hubiche T., Boralevi F., Thambo J. B., Taïeb A. Propranolol for severe hemangiomas of infancy. *N. Engl. J. Med.*, 2008; 358(24):2649-51.

[101] Sommers Smith S. K., Smith D. M. Beta blockade induces apoptosis in cultured capillary endothelial cells. *In Vitro Cell Dev. Biol. Anim.,* 2002; 38(5):298-304.

[102] Itinteang T., Brasch H. D., Tan S. T., Day D. J. Expression of components of the renin-angiotensin system in proliferating infantile haemangioma may account for the propranolol-induced accelerated involution. *J. Plast. Reconstr. Aesthet. Surg.,* 2011; 64(6):759-65.

[103] Routledge P. A., Shand D. G. Clinical pharmacokinetics of propranolol. *Clin. Pharmacokinet.*, 1979; 4(2):73-90.

[104] Stoschitzky K., Lindner W., Egginger G., et al. Racemic (R,S)-propranolol versus half-dosed optically pure (S)-propranolol in humans at steady state: Hemodynamic effects, plasma concentrations, and influence on thyroid hormone levels. *Clin. Pharmacol. Ther.,* 1992; 51(4): 445-53.

[105] Silber B., Holford N. H. G., Riegelman S. Stereoselective disposition and glucuronidation of propranolol in humans. *J. Pharm. Sci.,* 1982; 71: 699-704.

[106] Reddy I. K., Mehvar R. Chirality in Drug Design and Development. CRC Press; 2004.

[107] Lalonde R. L., Bottorff M. B., Straka R. J., Tenero D. M., Pieper J. A., Wainer I. W. Nonlinear accumulation of propranolol enantiomers. *Br. J. Clin. Pharmacol.*, 1988; 26(1):100-2.

[108] Johnson J. A., Burlew B. S. Racial differences in propranolol pharmacokinetics. *Clin. Pharmacol. Ther.*, 1992; 51(5):495-500.

[109] Zain-Hamid R., Ismail Z., Mahendra raj S., Shuaib I. L., Mohsin S. S. The Pharmacokinetics of Single Dose vs Steady-State Doses of Propranolol in Cirrhotic Malay Patients. *Malays. J. Med. Sci.*, 2002; 9(1):16-20.

[110] Zhou H. H., Adedoyin A., Wilkinson G. R. Differences in plasma binding of drugs between Caucasians and Chinese subjects. *Clin. Pharmacol. Ther.,* 1990; 48(1):10-7.

[111] Green W. H. Child and Adolescent Clinical Psychopharmacology. Lippincott Williams & Wilkins; 2007.

[112] Mcainsh J., Baber N. S., Holmes B. F., Young J., Ellis S. H. Bioavailability of sustained release propranolol formulations. *Biopharm. Drug Dispos.*, 1981; 2(1):39-48.

[113] Mansur A. P., Avakian S. D., Paula R. S., Donzella H., Santos S. R. C. J., Ramires J. A. F. Pharmacokinetics and pharmacodynamics of propranolol in hypertensive patients after sublingual administration: systemic availability. *Braz. J. Med. Biol. Res.,* 1998; 31(5):691-696.

[114] Duchateau G. S., Zuidema J., Merkus F. W. Bioavailability of propranolol after oral, sublingual, and intranasal administration. *Pharm. Res.*, 1986; 3(2):108-11.

[115] Cid E., Mella F., Lucchini L., Cárcamo M., Monasterio J. Plasma concentrations and bioavailability of propranolol by oral, rectal, and intravenous administration in man. *Biopharm. Drug Dispos.,* 1986; 7(6): 559-66.

[116] Bianchetti G., Graziani G., Brancaccio D., et al. Pharmacokinetics and effects of propranolol in terminal uraemic patients and in patients undergoing regular dialysis treatment. *Clin. Pharmacokinet.,* 1976; 1(5): 373-84.

[117] Amin O. S. Get Through MRCP Part 1: BOFs. CRC Press; 2008.

[118] Calès P., Grasset D., Ravaud A., et al. Pharmacodynamic and pharmacokinetic study of propranolol in patients with cirrhosis and portal hypertension. *Br. J. Clin. Pharmacol.*, 1989; 27(6):763-70.

[119] Taegtmeyer A. B., Haschke M., Tchambaz L., et al. A study of the relationship between serum bile acids and propranolol pharmacokinetics and pharmacodynamics in patients with liver cirrhosis and in healthy controls. *PLoS ONE*, 2014; 9(6):e97885.

[120] Olanoff L. S., Walle T., Cowart T. D., Walle U. K., Oexmann M. J., Conradi E. C. Food effects on propranolol systemic and oral clearance: support for a blood flow hypothesis. *Clin. Pharmacol. Ther.,* 1986; 40(4): 408-14.

[121] Liedholm H., Wåhlin-Boll E., Melander A. Mechanisms and variations in the food effect on propranolol bioavailability. *Eur. J. Clin. Pharmacol.*, 1990; 38(5):469-75.

[122] Tripathi K. D. Essentials of Medical Pharmacology. JP Medical Ltd; 2013.

[123] Albani F., Riva R., Contin M., Baruzzi A. Stereoselective binding of propranolol enantiomers to human alpha 1-acid glycoprotein and human plasma. *Br. J. Clin. Pharmacol.,* 1984; 18(2):244-6.

[124] Belpaire F. M., Wynant P., Van trappen P., Dhont M., Verstraete A., Bogaert M. G. Protein binding of propranolol and verapamil enantiomers in maternal and foetal serum. *Br. J. Clin. Pharmacol.,* 1995; 39(2): 190-3.

[125] Walle U. K., Fagan T. C., Topmiller M. J., Conradi E. C., Walle T. The influence of gender and sex steroid hormones on the plasma binding of propranolol enantiomers. *Br. J. Clin. Pharmacol.,* 1994; 37(1):21-5.

[126] Bowman S. L., Hudson S. A., Simpson G., Munro J. F., Clements J. A. A comparison of the pharmacokinetics of propranolol in obese and normal volunteers. *Br. J. Clin. Pharmacol.*, 1986; 21(5):529-32.

[127] Collett A., Tanianis-hughes J., Warhurst G. Rapid induction of P-glycoprotein expression by high permeability compounds in colonic cells in vitro: a possible source of transporter mediated drug interactions? *Biochem. Pharmacol.*, 2004; 68(4):783-90.

[128] Masubuchi Y., Hosokawa S., Horie T., et al. Cytochrome P450 isozymes involved in propranolol metabolism in human liver microsomes. The role of CYP2D6 as ring-hydroxylase and CYP1A2 as N-desisopropylase. *Drug Metab. Dispos.*, 1994; 22(6):909-15.

[129] Shand D. G. Pharmacokinetics of propranolol: a review. *Postgrad. Med. J.*, 1976; 52 Suppl. 4:22-25.

[130] Walle T., Walle U. K., Olanoff L. S. Quantitative account of propranolol metabolism in urine of normal man. *Drug Metab. Dispos.,* 1985; 13(2):204-9.

[131] Sowinski K. M., Burlew B. S. Impact of CYP2D6 poor metabolizer phenotype on propranolol pharmacokinetics and response. *Pharmacotherapy*, 1997; 17(6):1305-10.

[132] Nace G. S., Wood A. J. Pharmacokinetics of long acting propranolol. Implications for therapeutic use. *Clin. Pharmacokinet.*, 1987; 13(1):51-64.

[133] Walle T., Walle K., Mathur R. S., Palesch Y. Y., Conradi E. C. Propranolol metabolism in normal subjects: association with sex steroid hormones. *Clin. Pharmacol. Ther.*, 1994; 56(2):127-32.

[134] Alomar M. J. Factors affecting the development of adverse drug reactions (Review article). *Saudi Pharm. J.,* 2014; 22(2):83-94.

[135] Castleden C. M., George C. F. The effect of ageing on the hepatic clearance of propranolol. *Br. J. Clin. Pharmacol.*, 1979; 7(1):49-54.

[136] Tateishi T., Fujimura A., Shiga T., Ohashi K., Ebihara A. Influence of aging on the oxidative and conjugative metabolism of propranolol. *Int. J. Clin. Pharmacol. Res.*, 1995; 15(3):95-101.

[137] Ochs H. R., Grube E., Greenblatt D. J., Knüchel M., Bodem G. Kinetics and cardiac effects of propranolol in humans. *Klin. Wochenschr.,* 1982; 60(10):521-5.

[138] Cheymol G., Poirier J. M., Barre J., Pradalier A., Dry J. Comparative pharmacokinetics of intravenous propranolol in obese and normal volunteers. *J. Clin. Pharmacol.,* 1987; 27(11):874-9.

[139] Elliott W. J. Drug interactions and drugs that affect blood pressure. *J. Clin. Hypertens. (Greenwich)*, 2006; 8(10):731-7.

[140] Wood A. J., Feely J. Pharmacokinetic drug interactions with propranolol. *Clin. Pharmacokinet.*, 1983; 8(3):253-62.

[141] Herman R. J., Nakamura K., Wilkinson G. R., Wood A. J. Induction of propranolol metabolism by rifampicin. *Br. J. Clin. Pharmacol.,* 1983; 16(5): 565-9.

[142] Bai S. A., Abramson F. P. Interaction of phenobarbital with propranolol in the dog. 3. Beta blockade. *J. Pharmacol. Exp. Ther.*, 1983; 224(1):62-7.

[143] Sakuma T., Ohtake M., Katsurayama Y., Jarukamjorn K., Nemoto N. Induction of CYP1A2 by phenobarbital in the livers of aryl hydrocarbon-responsive and -nonresponsive mice. *Drug Metab. Dispos.,* 1999; 27(3):379-84.

[144] Stolerman I. P. Encyclopedia of Psychopharmacology. Springer Science and Business Media; 2010.

[145] Miller R. T., Miksys S., Hoffmann E., Tyndale R. F. Ethanol self-administration and nicotine treatment increase brain levels of CYP2D in African green monkeys. *Br. J. Pharmacol.*, 2014; 171(12):3077-88.

[146] Flockhart D. A., Tanus-santos J. E. Implications of cytochrome P450 interactions when prescribing medication for hypertension. *Arch Intern. Med.*, 2002; 162(4):405-12.

[147] Gervasini G., Caballero M. J., Carrillo J. A., Benitez J. Comparative cytochrome p450 in vitro inhibition by atypical antipsychotic drugs. *ISRN Pharmacol.*, 2013; 2013:792456.

[148] Yamada K., Yasuhara M., Yatsuzuka A., et al. Mechanisms of pharmacokinetic interaction between propranolol and quinidine in rats. *Chem. Pharm. Bull.,* 1992; 40(7):1876-9.

[149] Reimann I. W., Klotz U., Siems B., Frölich J. Cimetidine increases steady state plasma levels of propranolol. *Br. J. Clin. Pharmacol.,* 1981; 12(6):785-90.

[150] Griffin J. P., D'Arcy P. F. A Manual of Adverse Drug Interactions. Elsevier Science Limited; 1997.

[151] Kowey P. R., Kirsten E. B., Fu C. H., Mason W. D. Interaction between propranolol and propafenone in healthy volunteers. *J. Clin. Pharmacol.,* 1989; 29(6):512-7.

[152] Kobayashi K., Nakajima M., Chiba K., et al. Inhibitory effects of antiarrhythmic drugs on phenacetin O-deethylation catalysed by human CYP1A2. *Br. J. Clin. Pharmacol.*, 1998; 45(4):361-8.

[153] Mclean A. J., Skews H., Bobik A., Dudley F. J. Interaction between oral propranolol and hydralazine. *Clin. Pharmacol. Ther.*, 1980; 27(6):726-32.

[154] Hall S. T., Harding S. M., Hassani H., Keene O. N., Pellegatti M. The pharmacokinetic and pharmacodynamic interaction between lacidipine and propranolol in healthy volunteers. *J. Cardiovasc. Pharmacol.*, 1991;18 Suppl. 11:S13-7.

[155] Zhou H. H., Anthony L. B., Roden D. M., Wood A. J. Quinidine reduces clearance of (+)-propranolol more than (-)-propranolol through marked reduction in 4-hydroxylation. *Clin. Pharmacol. Ther.*, 1990;47(6):686-93.

[156] Vercruysse I., Belpaire F., Wynant P., Massart D. L., Dupont A. G. Enantioselective inhibitory effect of nicardipine on the hepatic clearance of propranolol in man. *Chirality,* 1994;6(1):5-10.

[157] Hunt B. A., Bottorff M. B., Herring V. L., Self T. H., Lalonde R. L. Effects of calcium channel blockers on the pharmacokinetics of propranolol stereoisomers. *Clin. Pharmacol. Ther.*, 1990; 47(5):584-91.

[158] Hibbard D. M., Peters J. R., Hunninghake D. B. Effects of cholestyramine and colestipol on the plasma concentrations of propranolol. *Br. J. Clin. Pharmacol.*, 1984; 18(3):337-42.

[159] Al-Meshal M. A., El-Sayed Y. M., Al-Angary A. A., Al-Dardiri M. M. Effect of oral activated charcoal on propranolol pharmacokinetics following intravenous administration to rabbits. *J. Clin. Pharm. Ther.,* 1993; 18(1):39-44.

[160] Branch R. A., Shand D. G., Wilkinson G. R., Nies A. S. The reduction of lidocaine clearance by dl-propranolol: an example of hemodynamic drug interaction. *J. Pharmacol. Exp. Ther.*, 1973; 184(2):515-9.

[161] Orlando R., Piccoli P., De martin S., Padrini R., Floreani M., Palatini P. Cytochrome P450 1A2 is a major determinant of lidocaine metabolism in vivo: effects of liver function. *Clin. Pharmacol. Ther.*, 2004;75(1):80-8.

[162] Wang B., Zhou S. F. Synthetic and natural compounds that interact with human cytochrome P450 1A2 and implications in drug development. *Curr. Med. Chem.*, 2009; 16(31):4066-218.

[163] Maskasame C., Lankford S. M., Bai S. A. Effects of propranolol on the disposition and negative dromotropic activity of diltiazem in the dog during multiple dosing. *Drug Metab. Dispos.*, 1993; 21(1):156-61.

[164] Silver J. M., Yudofsky S. C., Kogan M., Katz B. L. Elevation of thioridazine plasma levels by propranolol. *Am. J. Psychiatry,* 1986; 143 (10):1290-2.

[165] Markowitz J. S., Wells B. G., Carson W. H. Interactions between antipsychotic and antihypertensive drugs. *Ann. Pharmacother.,* 1995; 29 (6): 603-9.

[166] Ogu C. C., Maxa J. L. Drug interactions due to cytochrome P450. *Proc. (Bayl. Univ. Med. Cent.),* 2000; 13(4):421-3.

[167] Yoshii K., Kobayashi K., Tsumuji M., Tani M., Shimada N., Chiba K. Identification of human cytochrome P450 isoforms involved in the 7-hydroxylation of chlorpromazine by human liver microsomes. *Life Sci.,* 2000; 67(2):175-84.

[168] Ochs H. R., Greenblatt D. J., Verburg-ochs B. Propranolol interactions with diazepam, lorazepam, and alprazolam. *Clin. Pharmacol. Ther.,* 1984; 36(4):451-5.

[169] Ochs H. R., Greenblatt D. J., Friedman H., et al. Bromazepam pharmacokinetics: influence of age, gender, oral contraceptives, cimetidine, and propranolol. *Clin. Pharmacol. Ther.*, 1987; 41(5):562-70.

[170] Goldberg M. R., Sciberras D., De smet M., et al. Influence of beta-adrenoceptor antagonists on the pharmacokinetics of rizatriptan, a 5-HT1B/1D agonist: differential effects of propranolol, nadolol and metoprolol. *Br. J. Clin. Pharmacol.*, 2001; 52(1): 69-76.

[171] Peck R. W., Seaber E. J., Dixon R., et al. The interaction between propranolol and the novel antimigraine agent zolmitriptan (311C90) *Br. J. Clin. Pharmacol.*, 1997; 44:595–599.

[172] Miners J. O., Wing L. M., Lillywhite K. J., Robson R. A. Selectivity and dose-dependency of the inhibitory effect of propranolol on theophylline metabolism in man. *Br. J. Clin. Pharmacol.*, 1985; 20(3):219-23.

[173] Lombardi T. P., Bertino J. S., Goldberg A., Middleton E., Slaughter R. L. The effects of a beta-2 selective adrenergic agonist and a beta-nonselective antagonist on theophylline clearance. *J. Clin. Pharmacol.,* 1987; 27(7):523-9.

[174] Lesko L. J. Pharmacokinetic drug interactions with amiodarone. *Clin. Pharmacokinet.,* 1989; 17(2):130-40.

[175] Yoshiyama Y., Sugiyama T., Miyazaki H., Kanke M., Shimada H. Toxic interactions between disopyramide and propranolol in chick embryos. *Biol. Pharm. Bull.*, 1997; 20(12):1310-2.

[176] Nechwatal W., König E., Isbary J., Greding H. [Hemodynamic interaction of propranolol and digitalis in patients with arterial hypertension (author's transl)]. *Z. Kardiol.*, 1977; 66(10):572-7.

[177] Murdoch D. L., Thomson G. D., Thompson G. G., Murray G. D., Brodie M. J., Mcinnes G. T. Evaluation of potential pharmacodynamic and pharmacokinetic interactions between verapamil and propranolol in normal subjects. *Br. J. Clin. Pharmacol.*, 1991; 31(3):323-32.

[178] Bailey D. G., Carruthers S. G. Interaction between oral verapamil and beta-blockers during submaximal exercise: relevance of ancillary properties. *Clin. Pharmacol. Ther.*, 1991; 49(4):370-6.

[179] Belz G. G., Essig J., Erb K., et al. Pharmacokinetic and pharmacodynamic interactions between the ACE inhibitor cilazapril and beta-adrenoceptor antagonist propranolol in healthy subjects and in hypertensive patients. *Br. J. Clin. Pharmacol.*, 1989; 27 Suppl. 2:317S-322S.

[180] O'malley K., Velasco M., Wells J., Mcnay J. Mechanism of the interaction of propranolol and a potent vasodilator antihypertensive agent - minoxidil. *Eur. J. Clin. Pharmacol.*, 1976; 09(5-6):355-60.

[181] Rubin P., Jackson G., Blaschke T. Studies on the clinical pharmacology of prazosin. II: The influence of indomethacin and of propranolol on the action and disposition of prazosin. *Br. J. Clin. Pharmacol.,* 1980; 10(1): 33-9.

[182] Stevens J. D., Mullane J. F. Propranolol-hydrochlorothiazide combination in essential hypertension. *Clin. Ther.*, 1982; 4(6):497-509.

[183] Warren S. E., Ebert E., Swerdlin A. H., Steinberg S. M., Stone R. Clonidine and propranolol paradoxical hypertension. *Arch. Intern. Med.,* 1979; 139(2):253.

[184] Donnelly P. Nurse's Handbook of Combination Drugs. Jones and Bartlett Learning; 2008.

[185] Gandy W. Severe epinephrine-propranolol interaction. *Ann. Emerg. Med.*, 1989; 18(1):98-9.

[186] Salort-llorca C., Mínguez-serra M. P., Silvestre-donat F. J. Interactions between ibuprofen and antihypertensive drugs: incidence and clinical relevance in dental practice. *Med. Oral Patol. Oral Cir. Bucal.,* 2008; 13(11):E717-21.

[187] Eadie M. J. Clinically significant drug interactions with agents specific for migraine attacks. *CNS Drugs*, 2001; 15(2):105-18.

[188] Aronson J. K. Meyler's side effects of cardiovascular drugs. Amsterdam: Elsevier; 2009.

[189] Hawkins N. M., Petrie M. C., Macdonald M. R., et al. Heart failure and chronic obstructive pulmonary disease the quandary of Beta-blockers and Beta-agonists. *J. Am. Coll. Cardiol.,* 2011; 57(21):2127-38.

[190] Minton N. A., Baird A. R., Henry J. A. Modulation of the effects of salbutamol by propranolol and atenolol. *Eur. J. Clin. Pharmacol.,* 1989; 36(5): 449-53.

[191] Kawano Y., Abe H., Kojima S., Takishita S., Omae T. Effects of propranolol on cardiovascular and neurohumoral actions of alcohol in hypertensive patients. *Blood Press.,* 1999; 8(1):37-42.

In: Propranolol
Editor: Mislav Puljević

ISBN: 978-1-63482-974-8

Chapter 2

Propranolol Adverse Reactions

Marko Skelin, M. Pharm[1,*] and Eugen Javor, M. Pharm[2]
[1]General Hospital Sibenik, Medicinal Products' Safety Committee, External expert
[2]University Hospital Centre Sisters of Mercy, Zagreb

Abstract

Systematic review of propranolol adverse reactions will be presented in this chapter on the basis of all accessible data in scientific literature. The most common adverse reactions are due to known pharmacological properties of non-selective beta-blockade and propranolol high lipophilicity. Reactions that do not appear to be a result of beta-adrenergic receptor blockade are very rare. Abrupt cessation of chronic propranolol therapy can induce adverse reactions regarding exacerbation of angina pectoris and, in some cases, acute myocardial infarction. Propranolol overdose can lead to hypotension, bradycardia, bronchospasm and acute cardiac insufficiency. Recently, propranolol is approved for indication proliferating infantile haemangioma (IH) requiring systemic therapy in infants by Food and Drug Administration (FDA) and European Medicines Agency (EMA). Approval resulted in more common prescription of propranolol in this population following more available reports on adverse reactions for this indication. Common adverse reactions of propranolol regarding sleep disturbance, fatigue and gastrointestinal symptoms are reported in adult and pediatric population. However, lower respiratory tract infections such as bronchitis and bronchiolitis were reported only in pediatric population.

Keywords: Propranolol, adverse reactions, abrupt cessation, overdose, infantile haemangioma

[*] Correspondence: markoskelin@yahoo.com

Introduction

Propranolol has been in use in various indications for several decades. However, regarding pediatric population only approved indication till now is infantile haemangioma (IH) in 2014, thus in pediatric population it has been used off-label. Propranolol is a non-selective competitive antagonist of beta-adrenergic receptors, therefore, adverse reactions from known pharmacological consequences of beta-blockade are expected. Decrease in heart rate and blood pressure basically depends on $beta_1$-adrenergic receptors blockade and certain cardiovascular adverse reactions (e.g., atrioventricular conduction disturbance, congestive heart failure (CHF), bradycardia and excessive hypotension) may occur. Due to blockade of $beta_2$- adrenergic receptors certain cardiovascular, respiratory, endocrine and metabolic adverse reactions can appear (e.g., cold extremities, brochospasm, hypoglycemia and hyperlipidemia) [1]. Summarizing propranolol's adverse reactions from different studies is quite difficult because many factors may bias results. Results of well-done, randomized and controlled trials are considered better evidence regarding relative benefits of a drug. Observational study designs may provide important information for questions about tolerability and harms that is not available from controlled trials [2].

Adverse Reactions in Adults

Data on adverse reactions in prescribing information for propranolol of Food and drug administration (FDA) and in the summary of product characteristics (SmPC) of United Kingdom (UK) Medicines healthcare products regulatory agency (MHRA) have minor differences. EMA SmPC for propranolol tablets is not available at the moment so SmPC from MHRA will be used in this chapter, even though it is not representative agency for Europe because of national differences. Adverse reactions are summarized in Table 1 following prescribing information of FDA and SmPC of MHRA for propranolol tablets with immediate-release, extended-release, propranolol solution and injections, which are approved for label use in adults and geriatric population [3, 4]. Accessible data for variations in frequency of adverse reactions due to different pharmaceutical formulations are poor [3]. Seems that a method of administration of propranolol is also relevant regarding its adverse effects. A report from the Boston Collaborative Drug Surveillance Program documented more frequent adverse reactions after intravenous administration of propranolol [5]. Boston Collaborative Drug Surveillance Program study reviewed 800 hospitalized patients receiving propranolol. Incidence of adverse reactions was not dose depended, however, elderly patients were more prone to adverse reactions. Serious adverse reactions were documented in 10 (1.3%) patients corresponding to bradycardia followed by angina, shock, pulmonary edema and complete heart block. Adverse reactions are summarized in Table 2 [6].

Table 1. Adverse reactions of propranolol in SmPC (MHRA) and prescribing information (FDA)

System organ class	Adverse reactions		
	FDA prescribing information	MHRA SmPC	Frequency in MHRA SmPC
General		Fatigue and/or lassitude (often transient general	Common (1-9.9%)
		Dizziness	Rare (0.01-0.09%)
Cardiovascular	Bradycardia Congestive heart failure Intensification of AV block Hypotension Paresthesia of hands Thrombocytopenic purpura Arterial insufficiency, usually of the Raynaud type	Bradycardia Cold extremities Raynaud's phenomenon	Common (1-9.9%)
		Heart failure deterioration Precipitation of heart block Postural hypotension, which may be associated with syncope, Exacerbation of intermittent claudication	Rare (0.01-0.09%)
Central nervous system	Light-headedness, Mental depression manifested by insomnia Lassitude Weakness Fatigue Catatonia Visual disturbances Hallucinations; Vivid dreams An acute reversible syndrome characterized by disorientation for time and place, short-term memory loss, emotional lability, slightly clouded sensorium, and decreased performance on neuropsychometrics.	Sleep disturbances Nightmares	Common (1-9.9%)
	For immediate-release formulations, fatigue, lethargy, and vivid dreams appear dose-related	Hallucination Psychoses Mood changes Confusion Memory loss	Rare (0.01-0.09%)
Gastrointestinal	Nausea Vomiting Epigastric distress Abdominal cramping Diarrhea, Constipation Mesenteric arterial thrombosis Ischemic colitis	Gastrointestinal disturbance such as Nausea Vomiting Diarrhea	Uncommon (0.1-0.9%)
Nervous system		Paraesthesia	Rare (0.01-0.09%)

Table 1. (Continued)

System organ class	Adverse reactions		
	FDA prescribing information	MHRA SmPC	Frequency in MHRA SmPC
		Isolated reports of myasthenia gravis like syndrome or exacerbation of myasthenia gravis	Very rare (<0.01%)
Dermatologic	Stevens-Johnson Syndrome Toxic epidermal necrolysis Exfoliative dermatitis Erythema multiforme Urticaria	Purpura Alopecia Psoriasiform skin reactions Exacerbation of psoriasis Skin rashes	Rare (0.01-0.09%)
Hematologic and oncologic	Agranulocytosis, Nonthrombocytopenic purpura Thrombocytopenic purpura	Thrombocytopaenia	Rare (0.01-0.09%)
Ophthalmic	Dry eyes	Dry eyes Visual disturbance	Rare (0.01-0.09%)
Respiratory	Bronchospasm	Bronchospasm may occur in patients with bronchial asthma or a history of asthmatic complaints, sometimes with fatal outcome	Rare (0.01-0.09%)
Metabolic and endocrine	Hypoglycemia in neonates, infants, children, elderly patients, patients on hemodialysis, patients on concomitant antidiabetic therapy, patients with prolonged fasting and patients with chronic liver disease	Hypoglycaemia in neonates, infants, children, elderly patients, patients on haemodialysis, patients on concomitant antidiabetic therapy, patients with prolonged fasting and patients with chronic liver disease has been reported.	Very rare (<0.01%)
Allergic reactions	Hypersensitivity reactions, including anaphylactic/anaphylactoid reactions, pharyngitis and agranulocytosis Erythematous rash Fever combined with aching and sore throat Laryngospasm, and respiratory distress		
Autoimmune	In extremely rare instances, systemic lupus erythematosus has been reported		
Genitourinary	Male impotence Peyronie's disease		
Musculoskeletal	Myopathy, myotonia		

System organ class	Adverse reactions		
	FDA prescribing information	MHRA SmPC	Frequency in MHRA SmPC
Miscellaneous	Alopecia, LE-like reactions, psoriasiform rashes, dry eyes, male impotence, and Peyronie's disease have been reported rarely. Oculomucocutaneous reactions involving the skin, serous membranes, and conjunctivae reported for a beta-blocker (practolol) have not been associated with propranolol.		

Table 2. Patients included n=800, total adverse reactions n=78

System organ class	Adverse reactions	Number of patients affected	Frequency if defined
Serious adverse reactions			
Cardiovascular	Shock Bradycardia followed with angina Complete heart block	5 1 1	0,63% 0,13% 0,13%
Respiratory	Pulmonary edema	3	0,38%
Non-serious adverse reactions			
Cardiovascular	Bradycardia Hypotension Congestive heart failure or fluid retention 2:1 heart block	17 16 9 1	2,13% 2% 1,13% 0,13%
Central nervous system	Headache Dizziness Fatigue Tinnitus Blurring of vision Paraesthesias Depression	9	1,13%
Gastrointestinal	non specified	9	1,13%
Respiratory	Bronchospasm	4	0,5%
Dermatologic and sensitivity	Rash Fever	3	0,38%

Isolated case reports may reveal more information that are lacking in randomized controlled trials, particularly information about tolerability and harms [2]. The most common cause of propranolol's adverse reactions is due to known pharmacological properties of non-selective beta-blockade and high lipophilicity.

Cardiovascular Adverse Reactions

Propranolol decreases the chronotropic, inotropic, dromotropic, bathmotropic, and lusitropic response to beta-adrenergic stimulation. Therefore, certain adverse cardiac reactions may occur because of beta-receptor blockade [1] Due to decreased cardiac output worsening systolic heart failure and new heart failure can occur in patients who depend on high sympathetic activity to maintain cardiac output [7]. Also, due to variety mechanisms including a reduced cardiac output, occurrence of severe hypotension accompanied with syncope is possible [6]. Beta-blockade decreases a sympathetic activity and leaves unopposed parasympathetic activity, therefore, bradycardia may appear and also can increase AV conduction time [8].

Desai and associates reported an elderly patient with multiple risk factors for congestive heart failure (CHF) who developed severe hypertension. After administration of 20 mg hydralazin and 0.2 mg of intravenous propranolol, patient has developed pulmonary edema. Authors concluded that propranolol may precipitate acute heart failure in patients with compensated CHF [9]. Although propranolol should be avoided in overt CHF, it may be highly beneficial when used with close follow-up in patients with a history of failure who are well compensated and are receiving additional therapies [3].

There have been many reports on cardio respiratory arrest after oral administration of propranolol in cardiopulmonary compromised patients or in the case of an overdose. However, De Rover and associates published a case report in which an 18 year old healthy volunteer developed cardio respiratory arrest after a single oral dose of 80 mg of propranolol. Volunteer was active sportsman without any cardiac, pulmonary or physical disease [10].

Propranolol may produce cold extremities and could favor incidence of the Raynaud's phenomenon by causing a drop in cardiac output or by directly blocking beta$_2$-adrenergic receptors [1]. Considering patients with intermittent claudication, there is no enough evidence suggesting that propranolol adversely affects walking distance, calf blood flow, calf vascular resistance and skin temperature. Because of the lack of strong evidence, propranolol should be used with caution in patients suffering from peripheral arterial disease (PAD) [11].

Cardiovascular adverse reactions for propranolol in SmPC of MHRA and prescribing information of FDA and are summarized in Table 3 [3, 4].

Table 3. Cardiovascular adverse reactions for propranolol in SmPC of MHRA and prescribing information of FDA

<table>
<tr><th rowspan="2">System organ class</th><th colspan="3">Adverse reactions</th></tr>
<tr><th>FDA prescribing information</th><th>MHRA SmPC</th><th>Frequency in MHRA SmPC</th></tr>
<tr><td rowspan="2">Cardiovascular</td><td rowspan="2">Bradycardia
Congestive heart failure
Intensification of AV block
Hypotension
Paresthesia of hands
Thrombocytopenic purpura
Arterial insufficiency, usually of the Raynaud type</td><td>Bradycardia
Cold extremities
Raynaud's phenomenon</td><td>Common (1-9.9%)</td></tr>
<tr><td>Heart failure deterioration
Precipitation of heart block
Postural hypotension, which may be associated with syncope,
Exacerbation of intermittent claudication</td><td>Rare (0.01-0.09%)</td></tr>
</table>

Central Nervous System (CNS) and Nervous System Adverse Reactions

Central nervous system (CNS) adverse reactions may occur due to propranolol's high lipophilicity (it has great diffusion in tissues and crosses the blood-brain barrier) and decreased cardiac output [12]. Occurrence of CNS adverse reactions indicates that propranolol affects not only peripheral autonomic activity, but also some central nervous mechanism.

Several mechanisms may be implicated:

- blockade of central beta-adrenergic-receptors located downstream from, and at the terminals of, "vigilance-enhancing" central noradrenergic pathways
- blockade of central serotonin (5-HT) receptors
- centrally mediated non-specific actions on centrally located neurones due to the membrane-stabilizing effects of propranolol
- peripheral beta-blockade that induces changes in the autonomic activity in the periphery which are relayed to the CNS [13]

Parker reported a 63 year old patient who was receiving propranolol 160 mg/day for three months. His dose was increased to 240 mg/day because of increased frequency of anginal attacks. Within two days he developed agitation, excitement and combativeness. After reducing dose to 160 mg/day his symptoms disappeared [14]. Another case of a 42 year old woman who was treated with propranolol 80 mg/day for three months to control her hypertension, developed severe depression, marked apathy, social withdrawal and anorexia. Symptoms of depression diminished five days after reducing dose to 40 mg/day with resolution of symptoms in eight days [14].

Recently, Morrison and associates documented a patient who was receiving propranolol 160 mg daily for hypertension treatment and developed rapid eye movement (REM) sleep behavior disorder. Propranolol was reduced immediately by 20 mg every 3 days until stopped with consequently gradual withdrawal of the symptoms. The mechanism for this adverse reaction is unknown, but authors suggest that propranolol binding to 5-hydroxytyptamine receptors and decreased melatonin release may be implicated [15]. Pace-Schott and associates reported increased eyelid movements per minute in REM sleep during acute discontinuation of paroxetine and fluoxetine (i.e., selective serotonin reuptake inhibitors), supporting a serotonin link with REM sleep [16]. A relationship between propanolol binding to 5-hydroxytyptamine (5-HT) receptors and propanolol induced sleep disorder was documented. Mechanisms of sleep disorders are not known, however, authors documented that blockade of central or peripheral beta$_2$-receptors and/or central serotonin (i.e., 5-HT) receptors are in a relationship with the number of dreams, unlike blockade of beta$_1$-receptors where no significant relationship was observed [17]. Stoschitzky and associates documented decreased nocturnal production of melatonin with (S)-enantiomer of propranolol [18]. Therefore, it is possible that propranolol, through these actions, could induce abnormal behavior during sleep.

Robson described development of migraine after exposure to propranolol [19]. A stroke, as possible complication of migraine, was described in propranolol treatment in prophylaxis of migraine [20].

CNS adverse reactions for propranolol in SmPC of MHRA and prescribing information of FDA are summarized in Table 4 [3, 4].

Table 4. CNS adverse reactions for propranolol in SmPC of MHRA and prescribing information of FDA

System organ class	Adverse reactions		
	FDA prescribing information	MHRA SmPC	Frequency in MHRA SmPC
Central nervous system	Light-headedness, Mental depression manifested by insomnia	Sleep disturbances Nightmares	Common (1-9.9%)
	Lassitude Weakness Fatigue Catatonia Visual disturbances Hallucinations; Vivid dreams An acute reversible syndrome characterized by disorientation for time and place, short-term memory loss, emotional lability, slightly clouded sensorium, and decreased performance on neuropsychometrics.	Hallucination Psychoses Mood changes Confusion Memory loss	Rare (0.01-0.09%)
	For immediate-release formulations, fatigue, lethargy, and vivid dreams appear dose-related		

Gastrointestinal Adverse Reactions

Mild gastrointestinal (GIT) adverse reactions (e.g., nausea, dyspepsia, constipation, diarrhea) have been reported in 5-10% of patients [6].

Table 5. GIT adverse reactions for propranolol in SmPC of MHRA and prescribing information of FDA

System organ class	Adverse reactions		
	FDA prescribing information	MHRA SmPC	Frequency in MHRA SmPC
Gastrointestinal	Nausea Vomiting Epigastric distress Abdominal cramping Diarrhea, Constipation Mesenteric arterial thrombosis Ischemic colitis	Gastrointestinal disturbance such as Nausea Vomiting Diarrhea	Uncommon (0.1-0.9%)

Severe adverse reactions have been infrequent, though severe diarrhea, weight loss, dehydration and hypokalemia have been reported in scientific literature [21].

GIT adverse reactions are summarized in Table 5 [3, 4].

Respiratory Adverse Reactions

Respiratory adverse reactions occur, presumably, by unmasking parasympathetic and other bronchoconstrictor factors subsequent to propranolol blockade of bronchial beta$_2$-receptors [1]. Propranolol also promotes degranulation of mast cells and depresses central responsiveness to carbon dioxide (CO_2) [22].

Sloand and Thompson documented that intravenous administration of propranolol can induce pulmonary edema in patients suffering from pheochromocytoma but without clinical evidence of heart disease. Patient developed pulmonary edema after intravenous administration of propranolol. Authors suggest that mechanism causing pulmonary edema may have been a propranolol induced nonselective beta-blockade that led to unopposed alpha effects and sudden elevation of afterload [23].

Thus, propranolol is indicated as an adjunct to alpha-blocker in pheochromocytoma therapy [3].

Fraley and associates described three cases of severe bronchospasm and even one case of respiratory arrest in patients taking propranolol with no history of asthma or allergy. After discontinuation of propranolol and supportive bronchodilator therapy, bronchospasm was relieved [24].

Respiratory adverse reactions for propranolol in SmPC of MHRA and prescribing information of FDA are summarized in Table 6 [3, 4].

Table 6. Respiratory adverse reactions for propranolol in SmPC of MHRA and prescribing information of FDA

System organ class	Adverse reactions		
	FDA prescribing information	MHRA SmPC	Frequency in MHRA SmPC
Respiratory	Bronchospasm	Bronchospasm may occur in patients with bronchial asthma or a history of asthmatic complaints, sometimes with fatal outcome	Rare (0.01-0.09%)

Dermatologic Adverse Reactions

Beta blockers have the potential to worsen psoriasis lesions [1]. Propranolol induced psoriasiform cutaneous eruptions usually appear after long-term treatment (average duration of treatment is 10 months) [25].

Leukocytoclastic vasculitis (LV) was diagnosed in a 69 year old patient with medical record receiving glibenclamide-phenformin 2.5-25 mg/day and acarbose 50 mg 3 times/day for diabetes mellitus type 2 for the last ten years.

Table 7. Dermatologic adverse reactions for propranolol in SmPC of MHRA and prescribing information of FDA

System organ class	Adverse reactions		
	FDA prescribing information	MHRA SmPC	Frequency in MHRA SmPC
Dermatologic	Stevens-Johnson Syndrome Toxic epidermal necrolysis Exfoliative dermatitis Erythema multiforme Urticaria	Purpura Alopecia Psoriasiform skin reactions Exacerbation of psoriasis Skin rashes	Rare (0.01-0.09%)

Also, folic acid 5 mg/day, spironolactone 100 mg/day and propranolol 40 mg twice/day for alcoholic liver cirrhosis have been used for the last two years. After a diagnose of LV, propranolol was discontinued and gradual improvement of the symptoms followed. Iliopoulou and associates state that propranolol caused LV and related mechanism may be a manifestation of an immune complex disease [26].

Propranolol induced increased, exercise-related,, sweating in healthy volunteers probably due to an imbalance between beta and alpha-adrenergic activity. Thus, fluid-replacement regiment during exercise is recommended [27]. Dermatologic adverse reactions for propranolol in SmPC of MHRA and prescribing information of FDA are summarized in Table 7 [3, 4].

Metabolic and Endocrine Adverse Reactions

Hypoglycemia can occur in non-diabetic patients particularly those who undergo prolonged fasting or who are on maintenance dialysis [3]. Propranolol can mask adrenalin-induced symptoms of hypoglycemia (e.g., palpation, tachycardia, tremor) and diminish the rate of a rise of blood glucose toward normal level. [8] Sweating is only a mild symptom of hypoglycemia that is not typically blocked by propranolol, therefore may be more reliable diagnostic symptom. Hypoglycemia is probably developed due to propranolol blocking catecholamine-induced glycogenolysis, gluconeogenesis, and lipolysis [28].

Propranolol, by inducing peripheral vasoconstriction, will alter the lipoprotein lipase function which leads to triglyceride (TGL) plasma level increase and high density lipoprotein (HDL) reduction [29]. The importance of these effects in propranolol long-term treatment of patients with hypertension or ischemic heart disease is yet unknown. Although. it is known that high total serum cholesterol and low HDL concentrations are associated with increased risk for ischemic heart disease. [8] Propranolol is reducing basal metabolic rate and thermogenesis by beta blockade and can predispose to obesity [30]. Also, propranolol blocks beta$_3$-adrenoceptors which are responsible for increasing lipolysis, fat oxidation, energy expenditure and insulin action. It would be recommended, from theoretical point of view, to avoid propranolol in obese patients [31].

Hyperthyroxinemia has been reported in patients receiving high doses of propranolol (320-480 mg/day). According to authors, abnormalities seen in patients were due to drug-induced blockade of iodothyronine deiodination [32]. Metabolic and endocrine adverse reactions are summarized in Table 8 [3, 4].

Table 8. Metabolic and endocrine adverse reactions for propranolol in SmPC of MHRA and prescribing information of FDA

System organ class	Adverse reactions		
	FDA prescribing information	MHRA SmPC	Frequency in MHRA SmPC
Metabolic and endocrine	Hypoglycemia in neonates, infants, children, elderly patients, patients on hemodialysis, patients on concomitant antidiabetic therapy, patients with prolonged fasting and patients with chronic liver disease	Hypoglycaemia in neonates, infants, children, elderly patients, patients on haemodialysis, patients on concomitant antidiabetic therapy, patients with prolonged fasting and patients with chronic liver disease has been reported.	Very rare (<0.01%)

Genitourinary, Nervous System and Skeletal Adverse Reactions

Impotence in men has been documented after treatment with propranolol [33]. However, some authors suggest that certain bias may contribute to impotence. Aronson suggests that the cause of impotence is generally psychological in origin [8].

Case reports describe propranolol induced symptoms of myasthenia gravis in patients with no known history of defect neuromuscular transmission. This adverse effect seems to be dose independent, with reversal of symptoms after discontinuation of propranolol. Doses vary widely, therefore incidence is not dose depended. After discontinuation of propranolol, recovery follows [34-36]. Lipponi and associates reported carpal tunnel syndrome (CTS) in a 60 year old man who was treating hypertension with 120 mg daily of propranolol for 5 years. Discontinuation of propranolol gradually resulted with improvement of symptoms, demonstrating reversibility of the process.

Table 9. Genitourinary, nervous system and skeletal adverse reactions for propranolol in SmPC of MHRA and prescribing information of FDA

System organ class	Adverse reactions		
	FDA prescribing information	MHRA SmPC	Frequency in MHRA SmPC
Genitourinary	Male impotence Peyronie's disease		
Nervous system		Isolated reports of myasthenia gravis like syndrome or exacerbation of myasthenia gravis	Very rare (<0.01%)
		Paraesthesia	Rare (0.01-0.09%)

Authors suggest that median nerve compression by fluid retention, fibrotic reactions and vascular congestion may be implicated in the mechanism causing CTS [37].

Finsterer and Gelpi reported a 52 year old woman who was treating arterial hypertension with 30 mg of propranolol for 7 years. She developed mitohondrial disorder corresponding to double vision, myalgias, muscle cramps and hip and thigh muscle stiffness. Symptoms disappeared after propranolol discontinuation.

Thus, authors are suggesting that administration of propranolol may aggravate a mitochondrial disorder [38].

Peyronie's disease has been documented after treatment with propranolol [39].

Genitourinary, nervous system and skeletal adverse reactions for propranolol in SmPC of MHRA and prescribing information of FDA are summarized in Table 9 [3, 4].

Special Populations and Overdose

Pregnancy

Propranolol falls into FDA pregnancy category C (i.e., animal reproduction studies have shown an adverse effect on the fetus and there are no adequate and well-controlled studies in humans but potential benefits may warrant use of the drug in pregnant women despite potential risks). Propranolol crosses the placenta and can cause intrauterine growth retardation, small placentas and congenital abnormalities [3]. Propranolol reduces placental perfusion. This may result in intra-uterine fetal death, immature and premature deliveries. Bradycardia, hypoglycemia and/or respiratory depression were reported in neonates whose mothers were treated with propranolol at parturition [4].

Propranolol and propranolol glucuronide are detected in breast milk, but estimated infant daily dose derived from breastfeeding (less than 0.1% of the maternal dose) is too low to cause adverse reactions [40]. Nevertheless, breast feeding is not recommended during propranolol treatment [4].

Geriatric Use

Debelis and associates concluded that adverse reactions are common and often preventable among elderly patients in the ambulatory clinical settings, regarding all drugs in general [41]. Elderly patient liver has decreased ability to metabolize drugs and they have decreased ability of a kidney to excrete drugs into the urine. Also, elderly patients have more fat tissue and drugs that dissolve in fat accumulate more [42].

Because of those pharmacokinetic peculiarities in elderly people, propranolol metabolism is reduced and his accumulation is increased. Greenblatt and Koch-Weser reported more frequent propranolol adverse reactions in elderly patients, therefore, suggesting that geriatric population receiving propranolol is more prone to adverse reactions. Incidence of adverse reactions seems to be dose independent [6].

Abrupt Cessation

Abrupt cessation of propranolol may cause serious adverse reactions such as: exacerbation of angina, ventricular tachycardia, acute myocardial infarction (MI) and sudden death [43].

This increased risk is connected with upregulation of beta-adrenoceptors during a chronic treatment [44]. Propranolol should be withdrawn, gradually, over a period of 7 to 14 days [4]. Rangno and associates demonstrated that, before complete withdrawal of propranolol, prolonged administration of small dose prevents enhanced cardiac beta adrenergic sensitivity and other adverse events in hypertensive patients [45].

Drug Overdose

Acute overdose toxicity includes cardiac disorders (bradycardia, hypotension, heart bock, conduction delays, acute cardiomyopathy, asystole), neurological disorders (seizure, delirium, psychosis, depressed mental status, loss of consciousness, coma), respiratory depressant effect and bronchospasm [12]. General and supportive therapy measures (e.g., evacuating gastric content, glucagon, isoproterenol, dopamine and atropine) are recommended in case of an overdose with propranolol [3].

In the review, the American association of poison control centers in a 10 year period (from 1985 to 1995) and there have been 38 fatal cases where beta blockers were implicated as the primary cause of death. Propranolol had the greatest number of exposures (44%) and was suspected as the cause of death in 71% of fatalities, due to higher frequency of use over the time period studied and its greater toxicity. Adverse reactions in fatal cases correspond to dysrhythmias, bradycardia, asystole and cardiopulmonary arrest [46].

An overdose of 2060 mg resulted in death, although patient has survived a dose of 8000 mg [47, 48]. Jovic-Stosic and associates reported a 31-year-old woman which ingested approximately 3600 mg of propranolol along with ethanol. Poisoning manifests with coma, seizures, respiratory failure, hypoglycemia, circulatory shock and dysrhythmias. Propranolol is highly lipid-soluble beta-blocker so initiation of 500 ml intravenous of 20% lipid infusion followed. Improvement occurred after procedure [49]. Lifshitz and associates reported a case of a 16 year old boy who indigested 3200 mg of propranolol in a suicide attempt. A patient developed CNS depression and acute dilated cardiomyopathy 2 h after ingestion. Gastric lavage, activated charcoal, and mechanical ventilation followed. After echocardiographic examination, he was treated with isoprenaline hydrochloride and glucagon IV. Patient improved 12 h following treatment [50].

Scientific data describes correlation between dose and symptoms, respectively to seizures and QRS prolongation [51, 52].

Adverse Reactions in Pediatric Population

Propranolol is well studied in adults. However, reliable data of its use in infants and children are lacking. There is only 1 approved indication in pediatric population (i.e., IH) by FDA and EMA. In FDA prescribing information for propranolol tablets is stated that safety and effectiveness of propranolol in pediatric patients has not been established [3]. In MHRA SmPC is stated that propranolol is not intended for use in children [4]. Use of propranolol in pediatric diseases, except IH, is off-label. Recommendations for propranolol treatment of other pediatric diseases is based, in majority, on systematic review of case reports and case series, thus each institution design their own unique protocols [53-55].

Adverse Reactions in Infantile Hemangiomatreatment

Estimated incidence of IH is varying from 4% to 10% of infants. They mostly involute spontaneously but significant minority can cause morbidities and require treatment [56]. Adverse reactions in SmPC of EMA are from three clinical studies, including 435 patients with dosing 1 mg/kg/day and 3 mg/kg/day and maximum treatment duration of 6 months. The most common adverse reactions were non serious and they rarely led to discontinuation of medication.

Table 10. Adverse reactions in EMA SmPC and FDA prescribing information for propranolol solution

<table>
<tr><th>System organ class</th><th>Adverse reactions in FDA prescribing information</th><th>Frequency in FDA prescribing information for1.2 mg/kg/day N=200</th><th>Frequency in FDA prescribing information for 3.4 mg/kg/day N=224</th><th>Adverse reactions in EMA SmPC</th><th>Frequency in EMA SmPC</th></tr>
<tr><td rowspan="5">Cardiovascular</td><td rowspan="3">Second degree AV heart block in a patient with underlying conduction disorder</td><td rowspan="3">Not known</td><td rowspan="3">Not known</td><td>Peripheral coldness</td><td>Common ≥ 1% to < 10%</td></tr>
<tr><td>AV block</td><td>Uncommon ≥ 0.1% to < 1%</td></tr>
<tr><td rowspan="3">Bradycardia
Hypotension
Vasoconstriction
Raynaud's phenomenon</td><td rowspan="3">Not known</td></tr>
<tr><td>Peripheral coldness</td><td>8,0%</td><td>6,7%</td></tr>
<tr><td>Bradycardia
Hypotension</td><td>Not known</td><td>Not known</td></tr>
<tr><td rowspan="5">Central nervous system</td><td>Sleep disorder</td><td>17,5%</td><td>16,1%</td><td>Sleep disorder</td><td>Very Common ≥ 10%</td></tr>
<tr><td>Agitation</td><td>8,5%</td><td>4,5%</td><td rowspan="4">Agitation
Nightmares
Irritability
Somnolence</td><td rowspan="4">Common ≥ 1% to < 10%</td></tr>
<tr><td>Somnolence</td><td>5,0%</td><td>0,9%</td></tr>
<tr><td>Nightmare</td><td>2,0%</td><td>6,3%</td></tr>
<tr><td>Irritability</td><td>5,5%</td><td>1,3%</td></tr>
<tr><td>Metabolic and endocrine</td><td>Hypoglycemic seizure
Hypoglycemia, especially when children are not feeding regularly or are vomiting</td><td>Not known</td><td>Not known</td><td>Hypoglycemic seizure</td><td>Not known</td></tr>
</table>

System organ class	Adverse reactions in FDA prescribing information	Frequency in FDA prescribing information for1.2 mg/kg/day N=200	Frequency in FDA prescribing information for 3.4 mg/kg/day N=224	Adverse reactions in EMA SmPC	Frequency in EMA SmPC
Respiratory	Bronchitis	8,0%	13,4%	Bronchitis	Very Common ≥ 10%
	Bronchospasm	Not known	Not known	Bronchiolitis Bronchospasm	Common ≥ 1% to < 10%
Dermatologic	Urticaria Alopecia	< 1%	< 1%	Erythema	Common ≥ 1% to < 10%
				Urticaria Alopecia	Uncommon ≥ 0.1% to < 1%
Gastrointestinal	Diarrhea	4,5%	6,3%	Diarrhea Vomiting	Very Common ≥ 10%
	Decreased appetite	2,5%	3,6%	Constipation Abdominal pain Decreased appetite	Common ≥ 1% to < 10%
	Abdominal pain	3,5%	0,4%		
Still under investigations, not proven	Decreased blood glucose Decreased heart rate	< 1%	< 1%	Decreased blood pressure	Common ≥ 1% to < 10%
				Decreased blood glucose Decreased heart rate Neutropenia	Uncommon ≥ 0.1% to < 1%
	Agranulocytosis Hallucinations Purpura	Postmarketing report, not proven			
				Agranulocytosis Hyperkaliemia	Not known

However, a few rare cases of lower respiratory tract infections, like bronchitis or bronchiolitis, with an aggravation of symptoms (including bronchospasm) due to the bronchoconstrictive effect of propranolol are considered as serious adverse reactions. In the case of lower respiratory tract, infection associated with dyspnoea and wheezing, medication should be temporarily discontinued.

But in the case of reoccurrence and isolated bronchospasm, treatment with propranolol should be permanently discontinued. Cardiovascular adverse reactions were asymptomatic. During 4 hours of cardiovascular monitoring after drug initiation, a decrease in heart rate (average 7 bpm) and systolic blood pressure (less than 3 mmHg) has been reported. Propranolol can aggravate hypoglycemia in children, especially in case of fasting, vomiting or overdose [57].

Adverse reactions in prescribing information of FDA are from clinical trials with 424 patients included and treated with doses of 1.2 mg/kg/day or 3.4mg/kg/day for 3 or 6 months. Of these, 63% of patients were aged 91-150 days and 37% were aged 35-90 days at randomization [58].

Adverse reactions in EMA SmPC and FDA prescribing information are presented in Table 10 [57,58]. Infants in fasting state utilize glucose threefold higher, thus glycogen stores are lower and may give rise to develop hypoglycemia more easily [59]. Concomitant therapy may also bias hypoglycemia. Infants suffering from IH and treated with propranolol, may be at increased risk, developing hypoglycemia if they have received or are receiving concomitantly corticosteroids, due to adrenal suppression which may result in loss of the counterregulatory cortisol response [60]. Hypoglycemia, reported in infants, had strong bias because it was often associated with poor oral intake or concomitant infection. Cavalli and associates reported a tumor lysis syndrome (TLS) in a 33-day-old female who was receiving oral propranolol 2 mg/kg/day for IH treatment. She developed hyperkalemia and hyperphosphatemia 24 hours after starting medication. No treatment was required to reverse the TLS condition and the electrolyte alterations were mild, therefore the propranolol treatment was continued. Serum potassium and phosphorus levels diminished proportionally with involution of IH [61]. Data in scientific literature may explain symptoms of TLS. Malignant cells comparing to normal cells have fourfold-higher phosphorus content and high nucleic acid content [62]. Massive lysis of malignant cells induces hyperuricemia, hyperphosphatemia and hypocalcemia [63]. It is known that propranolol induces apoptosis in capillary endothelial cells in vitro and that abrupt breakdown of cells is a cause of hyperkalemia [64, 65]. Systematic review from 2013 included all studies (41 studies with a total of 1 264 patients) related to use of propranolol in IH treatment evaluating efficacy and adverse events of propranolol. Propranolol treatment was initiated on patients from 3 days to 10 years of age, dosing 1 - 4 mg/kg/day (majority was treated with 2 mg/kg/day) with treatment duration from 1 week to 15 months. In review, 74% of patients were female and 28% percent had received other medication (majority treated with oral prednisolone) before starting propranolol. Adverse reactions were reported in 39 studies on 1 189 patients within total 371 adverse reactions. Adverse reactions are summarized in Table 11. Serious adverse reactions were uncommon and rarely lead to discontinuation of treatment [56].

Review of a Consensus conference for initiation and use of propranolol for IH that was held in 2011, summarized all data on effectiveness and adverse reactions for IH treatment [28]. Historically, the burst of case reports and case series in IH treatment began in 2008 with the initial report of propranolol use in this indication by Leaute-Labreze and associates [66]. Limitations of accessible data are variability to the study design. Nearly all were retrospective studies. Thus, the true incidence of adverse reactions in IH population is difficult to determine and might be underestimated.

Table 11. Adverse reactions from systematic review. Patients included n=1189

<table>
<tr><td>System organ class</td><td colspan="2">Adverse reactions</td><td>Number of patients affected</td><td>Frequency</td></tr>
<tr><td rowspan="5">Cardiovascular</td><td rowspan="2">Hypotension</td><td>symptomatic</td><td>5</td><td>0,42%</td></tr>
<tr><td>asymptomatic</td><td>39</td><td>3,28%</td></tr>
<tr><td rowspan="2">Bradycardia</td><td>symptomatic</td><td>1</td><td>0,08%</td></tr>
<tr><td>asymptomatic</td><td>8</td><td>0.67%</td></tr>
<tr><td colspan="2">Acrocyanosis</td><td>61</td><td>5.13%</td></tr>
<tr><td>Metabolic and endocrine</td><td colspan="2">Hypoglycemia</td><td>4</td><td>0,34%</td></tr>
<tr><td rowspan="2">Central nervous system</td><td colspan="2">Fatigue
Insomnia
Nightmares
Night restlessness
Sleep disturbance</td><td>136</td><td>11,44%</td></tr>
<tr><td colspan="2">Irritation
Agitation
Behavioral changes</td><td>12</td><td>1,01%</td></tr>
</table>

System organ class	Adverse reactions	Number of patients affected	Frequency
Respiratory	Wheezing Bronchial hyperreactivity Bronchoconstriction Difficulty breathing Cough Bronchiolitis, Upper respiratory infection Stridor Pulmonary obstruction Cyanotic breath-holding spell	35	2,94%
Gastrointestinal	Gastroesophageal reflux Diarrhea Stomach upset Vomiting Poor feeding Constipation Viral gastroenteritis	41	3,44%
Other disorders	Benign infection	4	0,34%
	Rash	3	0,25%
	Exanthema/dry skin	3	0,25%
	Temporary hypotonia	3	0,25%
	Profuse sweating	2	0,08%
	Shaky	1	0,08%
	Streptococcal infection	1	0,08%
	Dental caries	1	0,08%
	Elevated alkaline phosphatase,	1	0,08%
	Ulceration	1	0,08%
	Hyperglycemia	1	0,08%
	Occasionally pale	1	0,08%
Not specified	/	7	0,59%

Table 12. Adverse reactions from review of Consensus conference. Patients included n=1175

System organ class	Adverse reactions		Number of patients affected	Frequency
Serious adverse reactions				
Cardiovascular	Bradycardia	asymptomatic and unknown	11	0,94%
		symptomatic	1	0,09%
	Hypotension	asymptomatic and unknown	33	2,81%
		symptomatic	3	0,26%
Metabolic and endocrine	Hypoglycemia		10	0,85%
Respiratory	Bronchoconstriction Bronchiolitis Wheezing Pulmonary obstruction Apneic episode		16	1,36%
Non serious adverse reactions				
Cardiovascular	Cold extremities		20	1,70%
Central nervous system	Sleep disturbance Nightmares		44	3,74%
	Somnolence		26	2,21%
Gastrointestinal	Gastroesophageal reflux disease or gastrointestinal upset		8	0,68%
	Diarrhea		9	0,77%

Table 13. Adverse reactions from RCT. Patients included n=19

System organ class	Adverse reactions	Number of patients affected	Frequency
Cardiovascular	Cold hands/feet	1	5,26%
Central nervous system	Sleep disturbance	2	10,52%
Respiratory	Bronchiolitis Streptococcal infection Viral upper respiratory tract infection	4 1 1	21,05% 5,26% 5,26%
Gastrointestinal	Viral gastroenteritis	1	5,26%
Other	IH ulceration Elevated alkaline phosphatase level Dental caries	1 1 1	5,26% 5,26% 5,26%

Adverse reactions from review of Consensus conference are summarized in Table 12 [28].

In a randomized placebo controlled trial (RCT) of propranolol for IH, 40 children between the age of 9 weeks and 5 years were included. Among 20 patients in propranolol group, 1 was excluded because of elevated liver enzymes, and in placebo group all 20 patients continued trial. Dosing regimen was 2 mg/kg per day divided 3 times daily for 6 months for propranolol group. Documented adverse reactions are summarized in Table 13 [67].

Adverse Reactions in other Pediatric Indications (off-Label Use)

Infants who received propranolol, for any indication, at the Children's Hospital of Wisconsin (CHW) from 2004 to 2011 and had an inpatient visit within 5 years after propranolol treatment initiation were included in retrospective review. There were 512 infants identified and received propranolol from whom 132 (63 female and 69 male) had inpatient visit and were included in a study. Age after propranolol treatment initiation ranged from 1 day till 12 months. Indications included were: arrhythmias, congenital heart disease, esophageal varices, hypertension and 1 case of IH. Dosing ranged from 0.23 mg/kg/day to 5 mg/kg/day with administration from twice till four times a day and duration of therapy from 1 day to longer than 6 years. Also, 87 patients had therapy duration longer than 1 month. Of 132 cases reviewed neither one hospital admission was identified regarded to adverse reaction, however serious adverse reactions were reported in 11 infants. Serious adverse reactions are presented in Table 14. All serious adverse reactions resulted in discontinuation of propranolol treatment, except hypoglycemia which had a strong bias. The serious adverse reactions occurred from 2 to 20 months after initiation of propranolol treatment, except for 1 patient, thus suggesting that adverse reactions may be delayed and not detected during hospitalization. Limitations of the study are related to its retrospective nature and reliance on the assumption that patients with serious adverse reactions will be readmitted to CHW. Another limitation is that patients had multiple coexisting medical conditions [53].

Isolated case report on an asymptomatic 7 years old female revealed another potential adverse reaction. Patient developed accelerated idioventricular rhythm (AIVR) due to propranolol treatment used for prophylaxis of supraventricular tachycardia (SVT). After discontinuation of propranolol, neither symptomatic nor asymptomatic arrhythmia was found. According to authors beta-blockade decreases sympathetic tone and heart rate and thus can cause AIVR [68].

Dental caries was developed in 2 patients with contributing factor of decreased salivation (beta blockade of salivary gland function), although formulation of the suspension (if it contains sucrose) may be bias in these reports [67, 69].

Table 14. Serious adverse reactions in retrospective review. Patients included n=132

System organ class	Adverse reactions	Number of patients affected	Frequency
Cardiovascular	Bradycardia	3	2,27%
Metabolic and endocrine	Hypoglycemia	1	0,76%
Respiratory	Bronchospasm Wheezing Asthma exacerbation	7	5,30%

A retrospective study at cardiovascular intensive care unit (CVICU) in Texas children's hospital included 241 patients with age ranged from 1 day till 18 years receiving beta blocker (atenolol, carvedilol, metoprolol and propranolol). The patients receiving propranolol were predisposed to have at least one adverse event. Adverse reactions were more common in pediatric population receiving beta-blockers in CVICU when comparing to pediatric population that is not in CVICU. According to authors, reason for higher frequency of adverse reactions among these patients is in fact that these children have less physiologic reserve [70].

Infants Overdose

Deaths or acute heart failure in pediatric population have been associated with propranolol initiation only in the settings of intravenous administration or drug overdose [46, 71].

A case of accidental overdose in a pediatric patient with a fatal outcome has been described in scientific literature. Patient's blood glucose level was 0 mg/dl, suggesting hypoglycemia, may be the most serious adverse reaction of overdose in children [46]. Reith and associates described two deaths from propranolol poisoning in pediatric population (ages 13 and 17).

Propranolol levels in serum were 3.8 mg/L and 2.9 mg/L and in liver 50 mg/kg and 47 mg/kg respectively [51].

Comparison

Certain adverse reactions are documented only in pediatric population. Labeled adverse reactions documented only in pediatric population are presented in Table 15 [57].

The exact reason why these serious adverse reactions are noticed only in pediatric population is still unknown.

Table 15. Adverse reactions from EMA SmPC reported only in pediatric population

System organ class	Adverse reactions	Frequency
Respiratory	Bronchitis	Very Common ≥ 10%
	Bronchiolitis	Common ≥ 1% to < 10%

Conclusion

Propranolol adverse reactions are in majority related to known pharmacological properties of non-selective beta-blockade and high lipophilicity. Propranolol is generally well tolerated and serious adverse reactions are rare. Adverse reactions usually involve cardiovascular, CNS, gastrointestinal and in pediatric population respiratory system. Also, elderly patients seem to be more prone to adverse effects of a propranolol. Serious adverse reactions are documented after abrupt cessation of propranolol, therefore it should be withdrawn gradually, over a period of 7 to 14 days. Although propranolol isn't often used as other beta-blockers in clinical practice nowadays, it has very well documented safety profile because of high frequency usage in past decades. Despite almost 50 years of propranolol presence in treatments of various diseases, there is still lack of data involving efficacy and safety of use in pediatric population. It was used off label in pediatric population until recently, when propranolol was approved for treatment of IH by FDA and EMA. It is realistic to expect increase in usage of propranolol in pediatric population and it is certain that further investigations in treatment of IH will reveal more information about safety of use in children. Bronchitis and bronchiolitis are reported only in pediatric population. Exact reason why these serious adverse reactions are noticed only in pediatric population is still unknown and needs to be more investigated before making any conclusion.

References

[1] Lechat P. Clinical pharmacology of beta-blockers in cardiology: trial results and clinical applications. *Hot Topics in Cardiology,* 2008;10:7-44.

[2] Helfand M, Peterson K, Christensen V, Dana T, Thakurta S. Drug class review: Beta adrenergic blockers. Update 4 [Internet]. Portland: Oregon Health & Science University; 2009 [cited 2014 Oct 1]. Available from: http://www.ncbi.nlm.nih.gov/books/NBK47172/

[3] Food and Drug Administration [Internet]. Maryland: Food and Drug Administration;2011 [cited 2014 Oct 2]. InnoPran XL (propranolol hydrochloride) Tablets Rx only; [about 5 screens]. Available from: http://www.accessdata.fda.gov /drugsatfda_docs /label/2010/021438s013s014lbl.pdf.

[4] Medicines and Healthcare Products Regulatory Agency [Internet]. London: Medicines and Healthcare Products Regulatory Agency; 2000 [updated 2011 Jan 20, cited 2014 Oct 2];Medicines Information; Inderal; [About 7 screens]. Available from: http://www.mhra.gov.uk/home /groups/spcpil/documents/spcpil/con1417760346231. pdf .

[5] Greenblatt DJ, Koch-Weser J. Adverse reactions to propranolol in hospitalized medical patients: a report from the Boston Collaborative Drug Surveillance Program. *Am. Heart J.,* 1973;86(4):478-84.

[6] Greenblatt DJ, Koch-Weser J. Clinical toxicity of propranolol and practolol: a report from the Boston Collaborative Drug Surveillance Program. A very G, ed. Cardiovascular drugs, vol 2. 1978;179-195.

[7] Thomas JA, Marks BH. Plasma norepinephrine in congestive heart failure. *Am. J. Cardiol.,* 1978;41(2):233-43.

[8] Aronson JK. Meyler's side effects of cardiovascular drugs. Amsterdam: Elsevier; 2009.

[9] Desai SP, Pierce EC, Fleming TC. Severe hypertension, propranolol, and acute pulmonary edema. *Crit Care Med.,* 1987;15(8):799-800.

[10] De Rover M, Van noorden MS, Nieuwenhuis S, Van der wee NJ. Cardiorespiratory arrest in a healthy volunteer after a single oral dose of 80 mg of the beta-blocker propranolol. *Neurobiol. Learn Mem.,* 2010;94(4):576-7.

[11] Paravastu SC, Mendonca DA, Da silva A. Beta blockers for peripheral arterial disease. *Cochrane Database Syst. Rev.,* 2013;9:CD005508.

[12] Dart RC. Medical toxicology. Philadelphia: Lippincott Williams & Wilkins; 2004.

[13] Koella WP. CNS-related (side-)effects of beta-blockers with special reference to mechanisms of action. *Eur. J. Clin. Pharmacol.,* 1985;28 Suppl:55-63.

[14] Parker WA. Propranolol-induced depression and psychosis. *Clin. Pharm.,* 1985;4(2):214-8.

[15] Morrison I, Frangulyan R, Riha RL. Beta-blockers as a cause of violent rapid eye movement sleep behavior disorder: a poorly recognized but common cause of violent parasomnias. *Am. J. Med.,* 2011;124(1):e11.

[16] Pace-Schott, E.F., Gersh, T., Silvestri, R. et al. SSRI treatment suppresses dream recall frequency but increases subjective dream intensity in normal subjects. *J. Sleep Res.,* 2001; 10: 129–142.

[17] Yamada, Y., Shibuya, F., Hamada, J. et al. Prediction of sleep disorders induced by beta-adrenergic receptor blocking agents based on receptor occupancy. *J. PharmacokinetBiopharm.,* 1995; 23: 131–145.

[18] Stoschitzky K, Sakotnik A, Lercher P, et al. Influence of beta-blockers on melatonin release. *Eur. J. Clin. Pharmacol.,* 1999;55(2):111-5.

[19] Robson RH. Recurrent migraine after propranolol. *Br. Heart J.,* 1977;39(10):1157-8.

[20] Bardwell A, Trott JA. Stroke in migraine as a consequence of propranolol. *Headache,* 1987;27(7):381-3.

[21] Robinson JD, Burtner DE. Severe diarrhea secondary to propranolol. *Drug IntellClin Pharm.,* 1981;15(1):49-50.

[22] Trembath PW, Taylor EA, Varley J, Turner P. Effect of propranolol on the ventilatory response to hypercapnia in man. *Clin. Sci.,* 1979;57 (5):465-8.

[23] Sloand EM, Thompson BT. Propranolol-induced pulmonary edema and shock in a patient with pheochromocytoma. *Arch. Intern. Med.,* 1984; 144 (1):173-4.

[24] Fraley DS, Bruns FJ, Segel DP, Adler S. Propranolol-related bronchospasm in patients without history of asthma. *South Med. J.,* 1980;73(2):238-40.

[25] Jensen HA, Mikkelsen HI, Wadskow S, Sondergaard J. Cutaneous reactions to propranolol (Inderal). *Acta Med. Scand .,*1976;199(5):363-7.

[26] Iliopoulou A, Giannakopoulos G, Synetos A, Georgiou A, Chalkiadaki A. Leukocytoclastic vasculitis: is propranolol implicated?. *Pharmacotherapy,* 2000;20(7):848-50.

[27] Gordon NF. Effect of selective and nonselective beta-adrenoceptor blockade on thermoregulation during prolonged exercise in heat. *Am. J. Cardiol.,* 1985;55(10):74D-78D.

[28] Drolet BA, Frommelt PC, Chamlin SL, et al. Initiation and use of propranolol for infantile hemangioma: report of a consensus conference. *Pediatrics,* 2013;131(1):128-40.

[29] Fogari R, Zoppi A, Tettamanti F, et al. Beta-blocker effects on plasma lipids in antihypertensive therapy: importance of the duration of treatment and the lipid status before treatment. *J. Cardiovasc. Pharmacol.,* 1990;16 (Suppl 5):S76-S80.

[30] Astrup A. Obesity and diabetes as side-effects of beta-blockers. *Ugeskrift for laeger,* 1990;152(40):2905--2908.

[31] De Souza CJ, Burkey BF. Beta 3-adrenoceptor agonists as anti-diabetic and anti-obesity drugs in humans. *Curr. Pharm. Des.,* 2001;7(14):1433-49.

[32] Cooper DS, Daniels GH, Ladenson PW, Ridgway EC. Hyperthyroxinemia in patients treated with high-dose propranolol. *Am. J. Med.,* 1982;73(6):867-71.

[33] A randomized trial of propranolol in patients with acute myocardial infarction. I. Mortality results. *JAMA,* 1982;247(12):1707-14.

[34] Herishanu Y, Rosenberg P. Letter: Beta-blockers and myasthenia gravis. *Ann. Intern. Med.,* 1975;83:834-835.

[35] Weber JC. Beta-adrenoreceptor antagonists and diplopia. *Lancet,* 1982;2(8302):826-827.

[36] Choi KL, Wat MS, Kung AW, et al. Phaeochromocytoma associated with myasthenia gravis precipitated by propranolol treatment. *Aust. N Z J. Med.,* 1995;25:257.

[37] Lipponi G, Lucantoni C, Antonicelli R, Gaetti R. Clinical and electromyographic evidence of carpal tunnel syndrome in a hypertensive patient with chronic beta-blocker treatment. *Ital. J. Neurol. Sci.,* 1992;13(2):157-9.

[38] Finsterer J, Gelpi E. Mitochondrial disorder aggravated by propranolol. *South Med. J.,* 2006;99(7):768-71.

[39] Osborne DR. Propranolol and Peyronie's disease. *Lancet,* 1977;1(8021):1111.

[40] Smith MT, Livingstone I, Hooper WD, Eadie MJ, Triggs EJ. Propranolol, propranolol glucuronide, and naphthoxylactic acid in breast milk and plasma. *Ther Drug Monit.,* 1983;5(1):87-93.

[41] Debellis K., Field T.S., Gurwitz J.H., Harrold L.R., Rothschild J., Seger A.C. Incidence and preventability of adverse drug events among older persons in the ambulatory setting. *JAMA,* 2003;289(9):1107–1116.

[42] Mangoni AA, Jackson SH. Age-related changes in pharmacokinetics and pharmacodynamics: basic principles and practical applications. *Br. J. Clin. Pharmacol.,* 2004;57(1):6-14.

[43] Miller RR, Olson HG, Amsterdam EA, Mason DT. Propranolol-withdrawal rebound phenomenon. Exacerbation of coronary events after abrupt cessation of antianginal therapy. *N. Engl. J. Med.,* 1975;293 (9):416-8.

[44] López-Sendón J, Swedberg K, Mcmurray J, et al. Expert consensus document on beta-adrenergic receptor blockers. *Eur. Heart J.,* 2004;25 (15):1341-62.

[45] Rangno RE, Nattel S, Lutterodt A. Prevention of propranolol withdrawal mechanism by prolonged small dose propranolol schedule. *Am. J. Cardiol.,* 1982;49(4):828-33.

[46] Love JN, Litovitz TL, Howell JM, Clancy C. Characterization of fatal beta blocker ingestion: a review of the American Association of Poison Control Centers data from 1985 to 1995. *J. Toxicol. Clin. Toxicol.,* 1997;35(4):353–359.

[47] Suarez RV, Greenwald MS, Geraghty E. Intentional overdosage with propranolol. A report of two cases. *Am. J. Forensic. Med. Pathol.,* 1988;9(1):45-7.

[48] Tynan RF, Fisher MM, Ibels LS. Self-poisoning with propranolol. *Med. J. Aust.,* 1981;1(2):82-3.

[49] Jovic-stosic J, Gligic B, Putic V, Brajkovic G, Spasic R. Severe propranolol and ethanol overdose with wide complex tachycardia treated with intravenous lipid emulsion: a case report. *Clin. Toxicol.,* (Phila). 2011;49(5):426-30.

[50] Lifshitz M, Zucker N, Zalzstein E. Acute dilated cardiomyopathy and central nervous system toxicity following propranolol intoxication. *Pediatric emergency care,* 1999;15(4):262-263.

[51] Reith DM, Dawson AH, Epid D, Whyte IM, Buckley NA, Sayer GP. Relative toxicity of beta blockers in overdose. *J. Toxicol. Clin. Toxicol.,* 1996;34(3):273-8. 63

[52] Weinstein RS, Cole S, Knaster HB, Dahlbert T. Beta blocker overdose with propranolol and with atenolol. *Ann. Emerg. Med.,* 1985;14(2):161-3.

[53] Kwon EK, Joachim S, Siegel DH, Drolet BA, Holland K. Retrospective review of adverse effects from propranolol in infants. *JAMA Dermatol.,* 2013;149(4):484-5.

[54] Aptiz C, Webb G, Redington A. Tetralogy of Fallot. *Lancet,* 2009;374:1462-71.

[55] Hochberg Z. Practical Algorithms in Pediatric Endocrinology. S Karger Ag; 2007.

[56] Marqueling AL, Oza V, Frieden IJ, Puttgen KB. Propranolol and infantile hemangiomas four years later: a systematic review. *Pediatr. Dermatol., 2013*;30(2):182-91.

[57] European Medicines Agency [Internet]. London: European Medicines Agency; 2014 [cited 2014 Oct 1]. Hemangiol:EPAR-Product Information; [about 20 screens]. Available from: http://www.ema. europa.eu/docs/en_GB/document_library/EPAR_-_Product_Information/human/002621/WC500166910.pdf.

[58] Food and Drug Administration [Internet]. Maryland: Food and Drug Administration; 2014 [cited 2014 Oct 2]. Hemangeol (propranolol hydrochloride oral solution); [about 5 screens]. Available from:http://www.accessdata.fda.gov/drugsatfda_docs/label/2014/205410s000lbl.pdf.

[59] Van Veen MR, Van Hasselt PM, De Sain-van der Velden MG, et al. Metabolic profiles in children during fasting. *Pediatrics,* 2011;127 (4):e1021-7.

[60] Breur JM, de Graaf M, Breugem CC, Pasmans SG. Hypoglycemia as a result of propranolol during treatment of infantile hemangioma: a case report. *Pediatr. Dermatol.,* 2011;28(2):169–171.

[61] Cavalli R, Buffon RB, de Souza M, Colli AM, Gelmetti C. Tumor lysis syndrome after propranolol therapy in ulcerative infantile hemangioma: rare complication or incidental finding? *Dermatology,* 2012;224(2):106–109.

[62] Locatelli F, Rossi F. Incidence and pathogenesis of tumor lysis syndrome. *Contrib. Nephrol.,* 2005;147:61–68.

[63] Cairo MS, Bishop M. Tumour lysis syndrome: new therapeutic strategies and classification. *Br. J. Haematol.,* 2004;127(1):3–1.

[64] Sommers Smith SK, Smith DM. Beta blockade induces apoptosis in cultured capillary endothelial cells. *In Vitro Cell Dev. Biol. Anim.,* 2002;38(5):298–304.

[65] Jona JZ. Progressive tumor necrosis and lethal hyperkalemia in a neonate with sacrococcygealteratoma (SCT). *J. Perinatol.,* 1999;19(7):538–540.

[66] Leaute-Labreze C, Dumas de la Roque E, Hubiche T et al. Propranolol for severe hemangiomas of infancy. *N. Engl. J. Med.,* 2008;358:2649–2651.

[67] Hogeling M, Adams S, Wargon O. A randomized controlled trial of propranolol for infantile hemangiomas. *Pediatrics,* 2011;128(2):e259-66.

[68] Ozdemir O, Ceylan Y, Koksoy AY, Aydin H, Gultekin A, Andiran N. Accelerated idioventricular rhythm associated with propranolol treatment in a child. *Cardiol. J.,* 2012;19(3):330-3.

[69] Girón-Vallejo O, López-Gutiérrez JC, Fernández-Pineda I, Méndez NA, Ruiz Jiménez JI. Dental caries as a side effect of infantile hemangioma treatment with propranolol solution. *Pediatr. Dermatol.,* 2010;27(6): 672–673.

[70] Britt J, Moffett BS, Bronicki RA, Checchia PA. Incidence of adverse events requiring intervention after initiation of oral beta-blocker in pediatric cardiac intensive care patients. *Pediatr. Cardiol.,* 2014;35 (6):1062-6.

[71] Litovitz TL, Schmitz BF, Matyunas N, Martin TG. 1987 annual report of the American Association of Poison Control Centers National Data Collection System. *Am. J. Emerg. Med.,* 1988;6(5):479–515.

In: Propranolol
Editor: Mislav Puljević

ISBN: 978-1-63482-974-8

Chapter 3

Propranolol Use in Cardiac Arrhythmias

Mislav Puljević
University of Zagreb, School of medicine, University hospital Center Zagreb, Clinic for cardiovascular diseases, Zagreb, Croatia

Abstract

In this chapter a medical therapy for cardiac arrhythmias will be presented. The main review will be based on the use of beta blockers in arrhythmology. Chapter will be based on few case reports where propranolol achieved good result after all other antiarrhytmic therapy failed. Recently released guidelines prefer new cardio selective beta blockers, so it seems that propranolol doesn't have important role in treating cardiac arrhythmias any more. But, there is few diagnosis where is propranolol potential shown. Sometimes non selective beta blocker can do better than new selective beta blocker. Typical mechanism of beta blocker (including propranolol) affect the heart conduction system is already shown in first two chapters.

Antiarrhythmic drugs are used to suppress abnormal rhythms of the heart (cardiac arrhythmias). Many attempts have been made to classify antiarrhythmic agents. The problem arises from the fact that many of the antiarrhythmic agents have multiple modes of action, making any classification imprecise. There are four main classes in the Singh Vaughan Williams classification of antiarrhythmic agents:

- Class I agents interfere with the sodium (Na^+) channel.
- Class II agents are anti-sympathetic nervous system agents. Most agents in this class are beta blockers.
- Class III agents affect potassium (K^+) efflux.
- Class IV agents affect calcium channels and the AV node.

Drugs that suppress beta-adrenergic signaling by competitively inhibiting agonist binding to beta-adrenergic receptors ("beta-blockers") have important antiarrhythmic properties. They differ from most other antiarrhythmic agents by not directly modifying ion channel function; rather, they prevent the arrhythmia-promoting actions of beta-adrenergic stimulation.

Beta blockers are often the first line of medications used in treatment of arrhythmias. Their role has been established in treatment of Supraventricular tachycardia (SVT) and Ventricular tachyarrhythmias. Beta Blockers are also used as prophylactic medications in SVT, VT and Sudden Cardiac Arrest survivors. They are important components of treatment in VT storms, Atrial Fibrillation, arrhythmias during pregnancy, arrhythmias associated with congenital heart disease, Long QT syndrome, arrhythmias in cardiomyopathies and post-cardiac surgery arrhythmias. The choice of drug, dose and route of administration depends on the type of arrhythmia and clinical presentation and demographics of the patient. Along with "standard" indications for beta blocker in cardiac arrhythmias, there are few interesting indications where non selectivity of propranolol showed advantage to other modern selective beta blockers, but main indication is prevention of malignant arrhythmias.

Electrical storm is an increasingly common and life-threatening syndrome that is defined by 3 or more sustained episodes of ventricular tachycardia, ventricular fibrillation, or appropriate shocks from an implantable cardioverter-defibrillator within 24 hours. The clinical presentation can be dramatic. Electrical storm can manifest itself during acute myocardial infarction or in patients with structural heart disease, an implantable cardioverter-defibrillator, or an inherited arrhythmic syndrome. The presence or absence of structural heart disease and the electrocardiographic morphology of the presenting arrhythmia can provide important diagnostic clues into the mechanism of electrical storm. Electrical storm typically has a poor outcome. The effective management of electrical storm requires an understanding of arrhythmia mechanisms, therapeutic options, device programming, and indications for radiofrequency catheter ablation. Initial management involves determining and correcting the underlying ischemia, electrolyte imbalances, or other causative factors. Amiodarone and β-blockers, (especially propranolol), effectively resolve arrhythmias in most patients.

Patients with implanted cardioverter defibrillator (ICD) often have justified ICD activations no matter if the indication for implantation was primary or secondary prophylaxis of sudden death. First line therapy in the prevention of recidivate ventricular arrhythmia in these patients is antiarrhythmic therapy, but if this is inefficient, arrhythmic substrate radiofrequency (RF) ablation is recommended. Ablation treatment is an accepted procedure in patients with ischemic heart disease, but it has rarely been used in patients with idiopathic and particularly polymorphic ventricular tachycardia (VT). It must be emphasized that acute ablation is relatively successful, but because of substrates progression, relapses of VTs are very frequent (35%) [1]. Therefore, antiarrhythmic therapy remains an important therapy after the ICD implantation, before, and often after RF ablation [2].

In this chapter we will see five cases in whom the prevention of recidivate VTs was achieved only by an old nonselective beta-blocker propranolol (dose 20 × 40 or 2 × 80mg).

Patient 1: a 52 years old woman with ICD implanted as a secondary prevention after out-of-hospital cardiac arrest caused by ventricular fibrillation. There was no structural heart disease, coronarography was normal, and there was only arterial hypertension in patient's history. QTc interval was within the reference range, there were no Brugada syndrome elements, and no sudden death in family history. During the first year after the implantation, ICD was activated for more than 10 times because of polymorphic VT in spite of medicaments therapy. On one occasion even an electrical storm occurred. After the implantation, bisoprolol maximum dose was given, and later in combination with mexiletine, which was stopped as a result of intolerance. Combination with amiodarone was used for a short period of time but with no effects. Only after bisoprolol had been replaced with propranolol, there were no tachycardias and ICD stopped activating. Since then the patient has been followed-up for 5 years.

Patient 2: a 56 years old man with no family or individual heart disease history, or any other serious disease. ICD was implanted as secondary prophylaxis after relapsing syncopes caused by VTs. The first therapy with amiodarone had not prevented multiple ICD activations, so it was replaced by a combination of bisoprolol and mexiletine. Despite the new therapy, ICD continued to activate for several justified occasions (5 times). Only after bisoprolol had been replaced with propranolol, ICD stopped activating. Since then the patient has been followed-up for 3 years. In the meantime, mexiletine therapy has been stopped (it is unavailable in Croatia), so now he takes propranolol only.

Patient 3: a 69 years old man with ICD implanted after relapsing sustained VTs. The patient had no structural heart disease or any signs of ischemia. Coronarography was normal. In spite of the maximum dose of bisoprolol in combination with amiodarone, ICD was reasonably activated on over 20 occasions. On 3 occasions, an electrical storm was detected. Arrhythmia could not have been controlled even by the combination of bisoprolol and mexiletine. Only the replacement of bisoprolol by propranolol led to a complete VT suppression. In the last 3 years, the patient has not had any ICD activation. In the meantime, mexiletine therapy has been stopped.

Patient 4: a 86 years old man. Two years ago, he had inferioposterior myocardial infarction with ST-elevation (STEMI) and a year after he was hospitalized for hemodynamically unstable VT. Slightly reduced ejection fraction (EF 45%-50%) was determined, caused by inferioposterior hypokinesia. Coronarography showed an old collateralized occlusion of the right coronary artery (RCA) and irrelevant changes on other coronary arteries. Sustained VTs repeated daily, despite the use of different antiarrhythmics: bisoprolol, lidocaine, amiodarone, and magnesium. After the temporary electrode had been placed, conversion was achieved by overdrive electrostimulation, but only occasionally. However, electrical cardioversion had to be done in most cases (6 times). Only the combination of propranolol and lidocaine in high doses managed to suppress VT. The patient had a successful RF ablation of VT with propranolol therapy only. During the 2 years of follow-up, he has had no arrhythmia. ICD has not been implanted.

Patient 5: a 60 years old man. After anteroseptal STEMI with severely reduced left ventricular systolic function, the patient developed frequent VTs that responded neither to combination of bisoprolol and lidocaine nor to overdrive stimulation. The use of amiodarone induced a remarkable extension of the QTc interval without suppressing arrhythmia. On most occasions, arrhythmia had to be stopped by electrical cardioversion (5 times). Only after using propranolol instead of bisoprolol, arrhythmia was completely suppressed. When propranolol had been cancelled, because of septic shock, VT relapsed. After the septic shock had been stabilized, ICD was implanted and propranolol was included to the therapy again. Further follow-up (1 year) has not recorded any ICD activation.

Electrical storm activates the sympathetic nervous system. Although extremely high levels of endogenous catecholamines have been documented during cardiac arrest, the current guidelines for advanced cardiac life support state that epinephrine or vasopressin should be used in cases of pulseless VT or VF. Epinephrine induces intense vasoconstriction by stimulating the a-adrenergic receptor and redirecting blood flow to the central circulation, thereby increasing coronary perfusion. Studies have shown increased rates of spontaneous circulation, coronary blood flow, and short-term survival after the administration of epinephrine. However, catecholamines are proarrhythmic and may exacerbate ventricular arrhythmias. Epinephrine makes the patient more susceptible to VF, contributes to myocardial dysfunction, and increases myocardial oxygen demand by stimulating the β-adrenergic receptor. The beneficial a-adrenergic effects of catecholamines on coronary perfusion pressure may be outweighed by the detrimental effects of the β-adrenergic receptor on VF susceptibility and by the increased demand for myocardial oxygen.

β-Blockers play a key role in the management of electrical storm. Their effects were discovered in the 1970s, when they were studied as therapy for acute myocardial infarction (MI). Propranolol consistently decreases the incidences of fatal VF during acute MI and sudden cardiac death after MI. Between beta blockers, results are better with the use of more potent β-blockers and those that antagonized both the β_1 and β_2 receptors. In patients with congestive heart failure, propranolol decreases sympathetic outflow more than does metoprolol, perhaps because β_2 receptors prevail in failing hearts. The lipophilic nature of propranolol enables active penetration of the central nervous system and the blockade of central and prejunctional receptors in addition to peripheral β receptors. Propranolol may effectively suppress an electrical storm even when metoprolol has failed. Therefore, propranolol is the preferred β-blocker,

Conclusion

In these cases, non-selective propranolol was more effective in suppressing severe VTs than newer selective beta blocker bisoprolol. Unlike bisoprolol, propranolol blocks both beta 1 and beta 2 receptors (20% of beta adrenergic receptors in the heart) and owing to liposolubility also penetrates into the brain [3]. Thereby, it can also result in the central inhibition of the sympathetic nervous system. The unique stability effect on the membrane of myocytes has also been described [4]. Previous studies showed that propranolol in combination with amiodarone offered the best prevention of VT relapses [5]. The reason why propranolol is not widely used in patients with cardiomyopathy is the lack of evidence-based data for these indications. Studies in patients with cardiomyopathy have recently been conducted using only newer beta-blockers (carvedilol, metoprolol, bisoprolol) [6]. It could be useful to conduct a modern study on propranolol, because propranolol possibly has more beneficial effect on the survival of patients than selective beta blockers. We can again see potential of propranolol in treating cardiac arrhythmias. The propranolol's age and non selectivity shouldn't be the reason to underestimate it.

References

[1] Yokokawa, M; Desjardins, B; Crawford, T; Good, E; Morady, F; Bogun, F; et al. Reasons for recurrent ventricular tachycardia after catheter ablation of post-infarction ventricular tachycardia. *J Am Coll Cardiol.*, 2013, 61, 66–73. doi: 10.1016/j.jacc.2012.07.059. [PubMed] [Cross Ref]

[2] Wissner, E; Stevenson, WG; Kuck, KH. Catheter ablation of ventricular tachycardia in ischaemic and non-ischaemic cardiomyopathy: where are we today? A clinical review. *Eur Heart J.*, 2012, 33, 1440–50. doi: 10.1093/eurheartj/ehs007. [PubMed] [Cross Ref]

[3] Kostis, JB; Rosen, RC. Central nervous system effects of beta-adrenergic-blocking drugs: the role of ancillary properties. *Circulation.* 1987, 75, 204–12. doi: 10.1161/01.CIR.75.1.204. [PubMed] [Cross Ref]

[4] Anderson, R; Ramafi, G; Theron, AJ. Membrane stabilizing, anti-oxidative interactions of propranolol and dexpropranolol with neutrophils. *Biochem Pharmacol.*, 1996, 52, 341–9. doi: 10.1016/0006-2952(96)00212-2. [PubMed] [Cross Ref]

[5] Eifling, M; Razavi, M; Massumi, A. The evaluation and management of electrical storm. *Tex Heart Inst J.*, 2011, 38, 111–21. [PMC free article] [PubMed]

[6] Chatterjee, S; Biondi-Zoccai, G; Abbate, A; D'Ascenzo, F; Casagno, D; Van, Tassell, B; et al. Benefits of β blockers in patients with heart failure and reduced ejection fraction: network meta-analysis. *BMJ.* 2013, 346:f55. doi: 10.1136/bmj.f55. [PMC free article] [PubMed] [Cross Ref]

In: Propranolol
Editor: Mislav Puljević

ISBN: 978-1-63482-974-8

Chapter 4

Propranolol Use in Heart Failure

Jure Samardzic, MD, PhD*
University of Zagreb School of Medicine, University hospital Center Zagreb,
Clinic for cardiovascular diseases,
Zagreb, Croatia

Abstract

Propranolol, a first generation nonselective beta blocker, has not been adequately tested in heart failure. Use of beta blockers in general was once absolutely contraindicated in patients with congestive heart failure due to their negative inotropic characteristics. Strong evidence of clinical benefit was shown in large randomized trials with several newer cardioselective beta blockers (bisoprolol, metoprolol, carvedilol, nebivolol) in patients with heart failure. These trials have made beta blockers a standard of care in treating chronic heart failure. Beta blockers do not show a class effect and propranolol is not recommended in heart failure. This chapter explains the rationale for the use of beta blockers in heart failure. It reviews scientific and expert literature dealing with this issue with a focus on trials investigating the efficacy and safety of administrating propranolol in different types of cardiomyopathies and heart failure. Using propranolol in certain conditions such as hypertrophic obstructive cardiomyopathy or co-existing uncontrolable ventricular tachycardias should be considered.

Keywords: Propranolol, beta blockers, heart failure, cardiomyopathy

Introduction

Heart failure is a common clinical syndrome associated with high morbidity and mortality [1]. It is caused by a spectrum of structural and/or functional cardiac disorders such

* Correspondence: Jure Samardzic MD, PhD. University of Zagreb School of Medicine. University Hospital Centre Zagreb. Kispaticeva 12. 10000 Zagreb. Croatia. Tel: +385 1 236 7467. Fax: +385 1 236 7512. Email: jure.samardzic@gmail.com

as myocardial infarction, arterial hypertension or valvular disease. It is a condition in which the ability of the heart muscle to supply the body with adequate blood flow to meet it's metabolic demands is reduced. *Cardiomyopathy* in broad definition is a disease of the heart muscle. As such, it affects not only the heart, but all organ systems as well. Heart failure is usually a chronic long-term illness. Despite significant improvements in the last decades in both pharmacotherapy and special medical procedures such as cardiac resynchronization therapy, ventricular assist device implantation and heart transplantation, heart failure continues to emerge as an enormous global health problem.

Rationale for Beta Blockers in Heart Failure

In an attempt to adjust for a primary deficit in cardiac output in heart failure, body utilizes neurohumoral mechanisms such as the activation of the sympathetic nervous system, renin angiotensin aldosterone system and increase in antidiuretic hormone, atrial and brain natriuretic peptides and endothelin [2]. With these mechanisms the body strives to restore cardiac output by expanding the extracellular fluid volume and increasing myocardial contractility and heart rate. The goal of the neurohumoral system activation is to maintain systemic blood pressure by vasoconstriction and redistribution of blood flow to vital organs. Sympathetic augmentation is one of the first responses to a decrease in cardiac output in both heart failure with reduced and preserved ejection fraction. It is an autonomic compensatory mechanisms used to preserve cardiac output in failing heart [3, 4].

Activation of these compensatory mechanisms increases the release and decreases the uptake of norepinephrine at adrenergic nerve endings in myocytes. Circulating catecholamines released by the adrenal gland also bind to the adrenergic receptors in the heart [5]. However, in the long run sympathetic hyperactivity leads to functional and structural changes in the heart. It causes negative remodelling, myocyte apoptosis and progression of myocardial dysfunction [6]. Furthermore, chronic overactive sympathetic nervous system may cause gastric ulcers, cancer, asthma, atherosclerosis, stroke and increase in blood pressure. The degree of sympathetic activation in heart failure patients can be reduced by effective and long term treatment and improve clinical outcome. The most important adrenoceptor in the heart is the beta$_1$ receptor. When activated, it increases the heart rate (positive chronotropy), conduction velocity (positive dromotropy), contractility of the myocardium (positive inotropy) and the rate of myocyte relaxation (positive lusitropy). Chronic stimulation of beta adrenergic receptors decreases the responsiveness to beta receptor. This occurs due to downregulation and desensitization of the beta receptor and its coupled signaling pathways [7-9].

In neurohormonal substudies of heart failure trials it was shown that angiotensin convertase enzyme inhibitors (ACEIs), angiotensin receptor blockers (ARBs) and beta blockers reduce sympathetic activity [10-12]. Blocking alpha adrenergic receptors did not bring clinical benefit in patients with heart failure. Therefore, activation of the sympathetic nervous system, both nonselective and cardiac selective, provides the rationale for the use of beta blockers in heart failure.

Beta Blockers in Heart Failure

Beta blockade upregulates myocardial $beta_1$ receptor density in patients with heart failure. This helps to restore the inotropic and chronotropic responsiveness of the myocardium and consequently improve its contractile function. Beta blockers have negative inotropic effect on the myocardium. The acute effect in patients with systolic heart failure is to apparently worsen the haemodynamic state by causing a decrease in left ventricular contractility and cardiac output. Beside from reducing sympathetic activity, benefits of beta blocker therapy in improving cardiac efficiency in heart failure is manifested in restoration of the population of $beta_1$ receptor with better contractile performance and prolongation of myocardial relaxation by reduction of the heart rate. Beta blockers reduce the level of circulating vasoconstrictors such as renin, endothelin and norepinephrine [13-16]. These hormones increase afterload and therefore, contribute to the progression of cardiac dysfunction. Beta blockers might reduce myocardial gene production of some of the inflammatory cytokines contributing to the development of heart failure [17, 18]. They affect left ventricular remodelling and improve function in regions of hibernating myocardial tissue by reducing oxygen consumption and increasing their perfusion with the prolongation of diastole [19, 20].

Beta blockers inhibit beta adrenergic receptors competitively. Inhibition of beta receptors can improve myocardial function by reducing the sympatomimetic overstimulation. The first evidences that blocking adrenergic receptors has beneficial effects in chronic heart failure were published in the 1970s with practolol and alprenolol [21, 22]. There are many beta blockers on the market with different charecteristics which make them more or less suitable and effective for different indications and clinical use. They are usually distinguished based on their cardioselectivity, intrinsic sympatomimetic activity and ability to inhibit alpha adrenergic receptors aswell. The difference in benefit between beta blockers with and without intrinsic sympathomimetic activity was seen in a meta analysis performed by Freemantle et al. on post myocardial infarction patients which showed that beta blockers without intrinsic sympathomimetic activity were better in reducing morbidity and mortality [23].

Chronic administration of beta blockers in patients with systolic heart failure has been shown to be beneficial in providing positive haemodynamic changes which result in significant increases in exercise capacity, left ventricular ejection fraction, cardiac index and a minor increase in arterial pressure. Beta blockers should usually be initiated in stable patients, dose gradually increased and used with caution in recently decompensated patients. The administration of beta blocking agents to patients with poor left ventricular function may result in clinical and hemodynamic deterioration. Imediate discontinuation of a beta blocker in heart failure acutization is needed especially in severely hypoperfused patients. Re-institution of treatment with a beta blocker should be attempted before hospital discharge when patients are hemodinamically stabilized.

Beta Blockers in Heart Failure – Randomized Controlled Trials

The evidence of reduced mortality in heart failure patients on a beta blocker is strong. This was shown in large trials with cardioselective beta blockers such as metoprolol, bisoprolol and nebivolol [24-26]. Carvedilol, beta blocker which inhibits alpha receptors as well, is also recommended for treating heart failure [1]. All four mentioned beta blockers showed their benefit in large randomized controlled heart failure trials. However, there are no large randomized trials which assessed benefit of other beta blockers in heart failure including a nonselective beta blocker propranolol.

Four large placebo controlled randomized trials: Cardiac Insufficiency Bisoprolol Study II (CIBIS II)[24], Carvedilol Prospective Randomized Cumulative Survival (COPERNICUS) [27], Metoprolol CR/XL Randomised Intervention Trial in Congestive Heart Failure (MERIT-HF)[25] and Study of Effects of Nebivolol Intervention on Outcomes and Rehospitalization in Seniors With Heart Failure (SENIORS)[26] randomized more than 10000 patients with heart failure to placebo or a beta blocker (bisoprolol, carvedilol, metoprolol succinate CR/XL and nebivolol, respectively). A very large proportion of patients were already on an angiotensin convertase enzyme (ACE) inhibitor or an angiotensin receptor blocker (ARB). Benefits of beta blockers were additional to those already on concomitant therapy for heart failure. These trials showed that treatment with a beta blocker can reduce heart failure hospitalization and mortality.

One large randomized controlled trial [Beta-Blocker Evaluation of Survival Trial (BEST)] with bucindolol [28], a beta-blocker with partial agonistic characteristics, did not show a significant reduction in mortality, though its findings were overall consistent with the mentioned trials. This implies that there may be clinically relevant differences between beta blockers in reducing mortality in heart failure. Another randomized controlled trial [Carvedilol or Metoprolol European Trial (COMET)] showed that carvedilol increased survival compared with short-acting metoprolol tartrate (different from the longacting succinate formulation used in MERIT-HF) [29].

Based on these trials, four beta blockers – bisoprolol, carvedilol, metoprolol and nebivolol are recommended in addition to an ACE inhibitor or ARB if ACE inhibitor not tolerated, for all patients with a left ventricular ejection fraction ≤40% to reduce the risk of heart failure hospitalization and the risk of premature death [1]. Generally, beta blocker dose should be titrated and gradually increased to the point of maximal tolerant and recommended dose (Table 1.).

Table 1. Recommended beta-blockers in heart failure - starting dose and maximal dose

Name	Starting dose	Maximal dose
Bisoprolol	1.25 mg o.d.	10 mg o.d.
Carvedilol	3.125 mg b.i.d.	25-50 mg b.i.d.
Metoprolol	12.5/25 mg o.d.	200 mg o.d.
Nebivolol	1.25 mg o.d.	10 mg o.d.

Selective versus Non-Selective Beta Blockers

Beta blockers do not show a class effect. There are few large randomized trials comparing different types of beta blockers in heart failure [29]. Few large studies exist outside of randomized trial settings that have examined whether outcomes vary in regards to different beta blockers in heart failure. As both $beta_1$ and $beta_2$ adrenergic receptors enhance adrenergic neurotransmission, some studies have explored whether nonselective beta blockade may inhibit cardiac sympathetic activity more effectively than $beta_1$ selective blockade. Newton and Parker have shown that the acute administration of metoprolol to patients with severe heart failure was associated with increased cardiac norepinephrine spillover [12]. In contrast, the administration of a nonselective beta blocker propranolol until similar hemodynamic end points were reached resulted in a small but significant reduction in norepinephrine spillover. This suggests that nonselective beta adrenergic receptor blockade may have favorable inhibitory effects on sympathetic outflow to the heart.

A large, population-based registry of over 20 000 patients with a recent hospitalization for documented heart failure suggest that prescription of a non-selective beta blocker is associated with a lower risk of thromboembolic events compared with the prescription of selective beta blockers. This was most prominent for the outcome of acute coronary events, where patients on nonselective beta blocker treatment experienced fewer events (HR 0.78, 95% CI: 0.65–0.93) [30].

Some beta blockers are efficiently removed from the circulation by hemodialysis whereas other beta blockers are not. A recently published study showed that patients (n=3294) initiating high-dialyzability beta blocker such as atenolol, acebutolol or metoprolol had a higher risk of death in the following 180 days compared to low-dialyzability group (n=3294) which included patients initiating bisoprolol or propranolol [31]. This implies that renal function should raise awareness on choosing optimal beta blocker and estimating the effect of a prescribed drug. This potentially important issue warrants further investigations.

Nonselective beta blockers or partially selective beta$_1$ blockers are associated with metabolic disturbances such as hypoglicemia and hyperlipidemia. Beta$_2$ blockade, particularly if combined with alpha blockade, is associated with an increased occurrence of sexual dysfunction. Propranolol is a lyposoluble nonselective beta blocker which posseses no intrinsic sympathomimetic activity and does not affect alpha adrenergic receptors. It has not been adequately studied in heart failure. It is known that nonselective beta adrenergic blockers competitively block response to beta$_1$ and beta$_2$ adrenergic stimulation. This results in decrease in heart rate, myocardial contractility, blood pressure and myocardial oxygen demand. Lipophilic beta blockers like propranolol and metoprolol appear in high concentrations in human brain tissue and are associated with side-effects such as insomnia, dreams and nightmares.

Use of non-selective beta blockers might worsen peripheral artery disease by increasing smooth muscle tone in blood vessels. It might also worsen chronic obstructive pulmonary disease or glucose metabolism. These characteristics and lack of good evidence go against the use of nonselective beta blockers such as propranolol in heart failure, even more because selective beta blockers are available and their use in heart failure is evidence based.

Propranolol Trials in Heart Failure and Specific Considerations

Studies on propranolol in heart failure are mostly old, small, non randomized and uncontrolled. Beta Blocker Heart Attack Trial [32] randomized 3837 patients with an acute myocardial infarction to propranolol or placebo. Patients between the ages of 30 and 69 years, with no contraindication to propranolol, were randomly assigned to receive placebo (n=1921) or propranolol 180 or 240 mg daily (n=1916) 5 to 21 days after admission to the hospital for the event. Survivors of acute myocardial infarction with compensated or mild congestive heart failure, including those on digitalis and diuretics, were included in the study. A history of congestive heart failure before randomization was present in 710 (18.5%) patients: 345

(18.0%) in the propranolol group and 365 (19.0%) in the placebo group. At an average follow-up of 25 months, compared to placebo propranolol significantly reduced total, cardiovascular, and sudden cardiac mortality and reduced the incidence of nonfatal myocardial infarction and all coronary events. Benefit was seen in all subgroups, including those with heart failure. The incidence of definite congestive heart failure after randomization and during the study was 6.7% in both groups. In patients with a history of congestive heart failure before randomization, 51 of 345 (14.8%) in the propranolol group and 46 of 365 (12.6%) in the placebo group developed congestive heart failure during follow up. In patients with no history of congestive heart failure, 5% in the propranolol group and 5.3% in the placebo group developed congestive heart failure. A retrospective subgroup analysis of Beta Blocker Heart Attack Trial was carried out in patients with arrhythmic events. Patients assigned to take propranolol who had left ventricular dysfunction achieved a greater benefit than those assigned to the placebo group. However, a greater incidence of drug withdrawal due to congestive heart failure was observed in those patients assigned to receive propranolol [33].

In 2001 Maia et al. published a prospective study in which 20 outpatients (10 male, mean age 56 +/- 12 years) with mean left ventricular ejection fraction of 28% were included [34]. They evaluated the effect of propranolol introduction (10-20 mg/day) and weekly dose increase to achieve a heart rate of 60 bpm, or a maximum daily dose of 120 mg. They found on average, that after treatment with propranolol there was a significant increase in left ventricular ejection fraction (by 52%), E wave deceleration time (by 62%) and effective ventricular filling time (by 38.5%). Two patients developed mild congestion which was controlled by increasing diuretic doses with no need to interrupt the protocol. Four patients had bradycardia-related symptoms and nine patients developed hyperkalemia.

Talwar et al. published a study in 1996 on 56 patients with dilated cardiomyopathy (aged 14–68 years) who were already on angiotensin converting enzyme inhibitor, diuretic and digoxin and were given an initial challenge of propranolol in gradually increasing doses [35]. Forty-four patients tolerated propranolol and received the drug for 6 months; 12 patients deteriorated after starting the drug with worsening of congestive heart failure and/or low output syndrome. The patients who did not tolerate propranolol had higher left ventricular end-diastolic dimension (73 ± 8 vs 66 ± 8 mm, $P < 0.05$) and severe mitral regurgitation was more common in this group. Hemodynamically, these patients had higher heart rate, higher right ventricular end-diastolic pressure, higher mean pulmonary artery pressure, higher mean pulmonary artery wedge pressure and left ventricular end-diastolic pressure (102 ± 16 vs 89 ± 12 beats/min, 15 ± 7 vs 9 ± 4, 39 ± 16 vs 31 ± 12, 28 ± 8 vs 21 ± 8, 28 ± 8 vs 22 ± 8 mmHg, respectively, $P < 0.01$). Patients which did not tolerate propranolol had a significantly lower cardiac index compared to those who tolerated propranolol well (1.9 ± 0.6 vs 2.5 ± 0.6 L/min/m^2, $P < 0.01$). Forty patients completed 6 months follow-up evaluation and underwent noninvasive and hemodynamic study again. There was a significant improvement in New York Heart Association class, cardiothoracic ratio and left ventricular end-diastolic dimension in those patients (68% vs 62%, 66 ± 8 vs 62 ± 7 mm, respectively, $P < 0.01$). The left ventricular ejection fraction rose from 23% to 35% during the follow up period ($P < 0.001$). Hemodynamically, there was a significant decrease in heart rate, right ventricular end-diastolic pressure, mean pulmonary artery pressure, mean pulmonary artery wedge pressure and left ventricular end-diastolic pressure (91 ± 14 vs 71 ± 5 beats/min, 9 ± 4 vs 5 ± 3, 32 ± 11 vs 22 ± 7, 25 ± 9 vs 17 ± 8, 21 ± 7 vs 14 ± 4 mmHg, respectively $P < 0.05$). The cardiac index rose from 2.3 ± 0.6 to 3.2 ± 0.7 L/min/m^2 ($P < 0.01$). The authors concluded at the end that propranolol in dilated cardiomyopathy was associated with significant intolerance (21.4%) and that those patients who tolerated propranolol well seemed to have long-term benefit on propranolol. Another study also showed that even very low doses of propranolol were known sometimes to precipitate severe heart failure in elderly patients with ischemia [36].

Hypertrophic cardiomyopathy is a genetically determined heart muscle disease mostly (60 to 70 percent) caused by mutations in one of several sarcomere genes which encode components of the contractile apparatus. Hypertrophic cardiomyopathy is characterized by left ventricular hypertrophy of various morphologies, with a wide range of clinical manifestations and hemodynamic abnormalities [37]. In broad terms, the symptoms related to hypertrnophic cardiomyopathy can be categorized as those related to heart failure, chest pain or arrhythmias. Patients with hypertrophic cardiomyopathy have an increased incidence of both supraventricular and ventricular arrhythmias and are at an increased risk for sudden cardiac death and embolic stroke. Symptoms including those of heart failure and chest pain are due to the combination of diastolic dysfunction, left ventricular outflow tract obstruction, mitral regurgitation and "small vessel" ischemia due to microvascular dysfunction. There have been no large randomized trials on pharmacologic therapies in hypertrophic cardiomyopathy. As a result, treatment strategies are based upon observational data and clinical experience which imply that the use of beta blockers might bring clinical benefit by several mechanisms. Slowing the heart rate to prolong ventricular filling, decreasing the oxygen demand and reducing myocardial contractility to reduce left ventricular outflow tract obstruction [38-40].

The use of beta blocker therapy in asymptomatic patients with hypertrophic cardiomyopathy is controversial. Some studies have shown that neither selective nor non-selective beta blockade causes significant reductions in exercise capacity in patients with hypertrophic cardiomyopathy on top of implementation of lifestyle changes [41]. In the absence of large randomized trials, the use of beta blockers is based upon the understanding of the pathophysiology of hypertrophic cardiomyopathy, characteristics of these drugs and clinical experience [37-46].

In hypertrophic obstructive cardiomyopathy beta blockers with non vasodilatative characteristics like propronolol are applied. Alternatives include a calcium channel blocker verapamil and disopyramide - class Ia antiarrhythmic drugs. It has been reported on adult patients with hypertrophic cardiomyopathy that propranolol reduces inappropriate vasodilation in about half of patients with abnormal blood pressure response to exercise. Some patients with a tendency to severe sinus bradycardia or hypotension on exertion tolerate propranolol better than beta$_1$ selective beta blockers. Non-vasodilating beta blockers titrated to maximum tolerated dose are recommended as firstline therapy to improve symptoms in patients with left ventricular outflow obstruction [37]. By consensus, patients with symptomatic left ventricular outflow obstruction are treated initially with non-vasodilating beta blockers titrated to maximum tolerated dose but there are very few studies comparing different beta blockers. Small and mostly retrospective studies conducted more than fourty years ago suggest that propranolol given orally can reduce and even stop resting and provocable left ventricular outflow track obstruction and provide symptomatic benefit [44-46] (Table 2).

Table 2. Observational studies on propranolol in left ventricular outflow obstruction

Study name	Number of enrolled patients	Mean follow up	Outcomes
Flamm et al. [44]	11	6.7 months	Significant symptomatic improvement in all but one patient
Adelman et al. [45]	21	2 years	Four patients with latent obstruction became asymptomatic. Of the 17 patients with resting obstruction, 7 improved, 2 were unchanged, 5 deteriorated and 2 died.
Stenson et al. [46]	13	17 months	Propranolol improved symptoms of heart failure
Frank et al. [47]	22	5 years	Symptomatic improvement by 58% to 100%

In a study conducted by Frank et al. [47] on propranolol in 22 patients with hypertrophic obstructive cardiomyopathy symptoms like dyspnea, angina, palpitations, dizziness and syncope improved by 58% to 100% on propranolol. Average propranolol dosage was 462 mg/d and mean follow-up was 5 years.

Propranolol, practolol and placebo were each administered to 16 patients in the first double-blind trial of beta blockade in hypertrophic cardiomyopathy (15 with hypertrophic obstructive cardiomyopathy) for a 4-week period. Propranolol lowered the frequency of angina and dyspnea while practolol (a relatively beta$_1$ selective drug with intrinsic sympathomimetic activity) had a lesser effect on clinical symptoms. It is possible that the bradycardic effect of beta blockers results in an increase in left ventricular end diastolic volume and a decrease in left ventricular outflow tract gradient in patients with hypertrophic obstructive cardiomyopathy. In eight patients with hypertrophic obstructive cardiomyopathy propranolol or practolol lowered left ventricular end diastolic pressure despite an increase in left ventricular end diastolic volume. This suggests that an improvement in left ventricular relaxation has been achieved. Another study performed by Speiser and Krayenbuehl found no change in the diastolic pressure volume relation after propranolol was given to nine patients with hypertrophic obstructive cardiomyopathy [35]. Hess et al. observed that left ventricular end diastolic pressure and chamber stiffness were unchanged on propranolol. The time constant of isovolumic relaxation increased because beta adrenergic stimulation accelerates left ventricular relaxation in normal heart muscle and in hypertrophic cardiomyopathy [42].

Takotsubo cardiomyopathy is a transient cardiac syndrome that involves left ventricular apical akinesis and presents clinically as acute coronary syndrome. It was first described in Japan in 1990 by Sato et al. [48]. Patients often present with chest pain, have ST-segment elevation on electrocardiogram and elevated cardiac enzyme levels consistent with a myocardial infarction. However, when the patient undergoes cardiac angiography, no significant coronary artery disease is found and left ventricular apical ballooning is present. The Japanese word *takotsubo* translates to "octopus pot," resembling the shape of the left ventricle during systole on imaging studies. Although the exact etiology is still unknown, the syndrome is usually encountered in women and is triggered by a significant emotional or physical excitation. Pretreatment with propranolol and metoprolol in a study on 69 rats with experimental model of isoproterenol induced takotsubo cardiomyopathy showed improved survival to 90% and 100% respectively, compared with 60% in the isoproterenol group. Pretreatment with a beta blocker did not reduce the incidence and extent of akinesis or the structural damage showed by echocardiography and histology [49]. Another study showed that intravenous propranolol might be useful for treating dynamic microvascular obstruction in patients with transient left ventricular apical ballooning [50].

Arrhythmogenic right ventricular dysplasia (ARVD) is a disorder in which myocardial tissue is replaced by fibrous and fatty tissue. This disorder usually involves the right ventricle but the left ventricle may also be affected. The exact prevalence of ARVD is unknown. It is one of the most frequent causes of sudden cardiac death in young, especially athletes. Because of the progressive nature of the disorder, patients may present with any number of symptoms. One of the major goals in treating ARVD is to prevent sudden cardiac death. No drug has been shown to be completely effective in controlling or/and stopping the arrhythmias. Drugs used to prevent arrhythmias include: class III antiarrhythmic drugs sotalol and amiodarone, class II drugs (beta blockers) like propranolol alone or in combination with class Ia drugs procainamide, class Ic drugs flecainide or propafenone.

Patients with cardiomyopathies and heart failure have an increased risk for sudden cardiac death due to ventricular tachycardia and/or ventricular fibrillation. Not all beta blockers are equally protective for arrythmias. Hydrophilic beta blockers like atenolol are not as good as lipophilic beta blockers such as propranolol or bisoprolol. In addition to beta adrenoceptor blocking effect propranolol increases the threshold for ventricular fibrillation. The usefulnes of propranolol in controlling cardiac arrhythmias is discussed in this book separately.

Conclusion

Propranolol has not been adequately tested in heart failure in large randomized trials. Beta blockers with strong effect on $beta_1$ adrenergic receptors should be used in this setting. Beta blockers do not show a class effect and previously published trials on propranolol showed that it may even worsen heart failure. Propranolol might be considered as an option in certain conditions and circumstances such as hypertrophic obstructive cardiomyopathy or ventricular tachycardias with a dose titrated to a heart rate between 50 and 60 bpm.

References

[1] McMurray JJ et al. ESC Committee for Practice Guidelines. ESC Guidelines for the diagnosis and treatment of acute and chronic heart failure 2012: The Task Force for theDiagnosis and Treatment of Acute and Chronic Heart Failure 2012 of the European Society of Cardiology. Developed in collaboration with the Heart Failure Association (HFA) of the ESC. *Eur Heart J.* 2012;33(14):1787-847.

[2] Francis GS, Goldsmith SR, Levine TB et al. *Ann Intern Med* 1984;101(3):370-7.

[3] Floras JS. Clinical aspects of sympathetic activation and parasympathetic withdrawal in heart failure. *J Am Coll Cardiol.* 1993;22:72A-84A.

[4] Aggarwal A, Esler MD, Socratous F, Kaye DM. Evidence for functional presynaptic alpha-2 adrenoceptors and their down-regulation in human heart failure. *J Am Coll Cardiol.* 2001;37(5):1246-51.

[5] Fowler MB, Laser JA, Hopkins GL, Minobe W, Bristow MR. Assessment of the β-adrenergic receptor pathway on the intact failing human heart: progressive receptor down regulation and subsensitivity to agonist response. *Circulation.*1986;74:1291–1301.

[6] Nozawa T, Igawa A, Yoshida N, Maeda M, Inoue M, Yamamura Y, Asanoi H, Inoue H. Dual-tracer assessment of coupling between cardiac sympathetic neuronal function and downregulation of beta-receptors during development of hypertensive heart failure of rats. *Circulation.* 1998;97(23):2359-67.

[7] Bristow MR, Ginsburg R, Minobe W, Cubicciotti RS, Sageman WS, Lurie K, Billingham ME, Harrison DC, Stinson EB. Decreased catecholamine sensitivity and beta-adrenergic-receptor density in failing human hearts. *N Engl J Med.* 1982;307(4):205-11.

[8] Packer M. The neurohormonal hypothesis: a theory to explain the mechanism of disease progression in heart failure. *J Am Coll Cardiol.* 1992;20(1):248-54.

[9] Bristow MR, Minobe WA, Raynolds MV, Port JD, Rasmussen R, Ray PE, Feldman AM. Reduced beta 1 receptor messenger RNA abundance in the failing human heart. *J Clin Invest.* 1993;92(6):2737-45.

[10] The SOLVD Investigators. Effect of enalapril on survival in patients with reduced left ventricular ejection fractions and congestive heart failure. *N Engl J Med.* 1991;325(5):293-302.

[11] Sigurdsson A, Amtorp O, Gundersen T, Nilsson B, Remes J, Swedberg K. Neurohormonal activation in patients with mild or moderately severe congestive heart failure and effects of ramipril. The Ramipril Trial Study Group. *Br Heart J.* 1994;72(5):422-7.

[12] Newton GE, Parker JD. Acute effects of beta 1-selective and nonselective beta-adrenergic receptor blockade on cardiac sympathetic activity in congestive heart failure. *Circulation.* 1996;94(3):353-8.

[13] Yoshikawa T, Handa S, Anzai T, Nishimura H, Baba A, Akaishi M, Mitamura H, Ogawa S. Early reduction of neurohumoral factors plays a key role in mediating the efficacy of beta-blocker therapy for congestive heart failure. *Am Heart J.* 1996;131(2):329-36.

[14] Eichhorn EJ, McGhie AL, Bedotto JB, Corbett JR, Malloy CR, Hatfield BA, Deitchman D, Willard JE, Grayburn PA. Effects of bucindolol on neurohormonal activation in congestive heart failure. *Am J Cardiol.* 1991;67(1):67-73.

[15] The RESOLVD Investigators. Effects of metoprolol CR in patients with ischemic and dilated cardiomyopathy : the randomized evaluation of strategies for left ventricular dysfunction pilot study. *Circulation.* 2000;101(4):378-84.

[16] Krum H, Gu A, Wilshire-Clement M, Sackner-Bernstein J, Goldsmith R, Medina N, Yushak M, Miller M, Packer M. Changes in plasma endothelin-1 levels reflect clinical response to beta-blockade in chronic heart failure. *Am Heart J.* 1996;131(2):337-41.

[17] Murray DR, Prabhu SD, Chandrasekar B. Chronic beta-adrenergic stimulation induces myocardial proinflammatory cytokine expression. *Circulation.* 2000;101(20):2338-41.

[18] Ohtsuka T, Hamada M, Hiasa G, Sasaki O, Suzuki M, Hara Y, Shigematsu Y, Hiwada K. Effect of beta-blockers on circulating levels of inflammatory and anti-inflammatory cytokines in patients with dilated cardiomyopathy. *J Am Coll Cardiol.* 2001;37(2):412-7.

[19] Prabhu SD, Chandrasekar B, Murray DR, Freeman GL. Beta-adrenergic blockade in developing heart failure: effects on myocardial inflammatory cytokines, nitric oxide, and remodeling. *Circulation.* 2000;101(17):2103-9.

[20] Cleland JG, Pennell DJ, Ray SG, Coats AJ, Macfarlane PW, Murray GD, Mule JD, Vered Z, Lahiri A, Carvedilol hibernating reversible ischaemia trial: marker of success investigators. Myocardial viability as a determinant of the ejection fraction response to carvedilol in patients with heart failure (CHRISTMAS trial): randomised controlled trial. *Lancet.* 2003;362(9377):14-21.

[21] Waagstein F, Hjalmarson A C, Wasir HS. Apex cardiogram and sistolic time intervals in acute myocardial infarction and effects of practolol. *Br Heart J.* 1974;36(11):1109-21.

[22] Waagstein F, Hjalmarson A, Varnauskas E, Wallentin I. Effect of chronic beta-adrenergic receptor blockade in congestive cardiomyopathy. *Br Heart J.* 1975;37(10):1022-36.

[23] Freemantle N, Cleland J, Young P, Mason J, Harrison J. Beta blockade after myocardial infarction: systematic review and meta regression analysis. *BMJ.* 1999;318(7200):1730-7.

[24] The Cardiac Insufficiency Bisoprolol Study II (CIBIS-II): a randomised trial. Lancet. 1999;353(9146):9-13.

[25] Hjalmarson A, Goldstein S, Fagerberg B, Wedel H, Waagstein F, Kjekshus J, Wikstrand J, El Allaf D, Vitovec J, Aldershvile J, Halinen M, Dietz R, Neuhaus KL, Janosi A, Thorgeirsson G, Dunselman PH, Gullestad L, Kuch J, Herlitz J, Rickenbacher P, Ball S, Gottlieb S, Deedwania P. Effects of controlled-release metoprolol on total mortality, hospitalizations, and well-being in patients with heart failure: the Metoprolol CR/XL Randomized Intervention. Trial in congestive heart failure (MERIT-HF). MERIT-HF Study Group. *JAMA.* 2000;283(10):1295-302.

[26] Flather MD, Shibata MC, Coats AJ, Van Veldhuisen DJ, Parkhomenko A, Borbola J, Cohen-Solal A, Dumitrascu D, Ferrari R, Lechat P, Soler-Soler J, Tavazzi L, Spinarova L, Toman J, Bohm M, Anker SD, Thompson SG, Poole-Wilson PA. Randomized trial to determine the effect of nebivolol on mortality and cardiovascular hospital admission in elderly patients with heart failure (SENIORS). *Eur Heart J.* 2005;26(3):215-25.

[27] Packer M, Fowler MB, Roecker EB, Coats AJ, Katus HA, Krum H, Mohacsi P, Rouleau JL, Tendera M, Staiger C, Holcslaw TL, Amann-Zalan I, DeMets DL. Effect of carvedilol on the morbidity of patients with severe chronic heart failure: results of the carvedilol prospective randomized cumulative survival (COPERNICUS) study. *Circulation.* 2002;106(17):2194-9.

[28] Beta-Blocker Evaluation of Survival Trial Investigators. A trial of the beta-blocker bucindolol in patients with advanced chronic heart failure. *N Engl J Med.* 2001;344(22):1659-67.

[29] Poole-Wilson PA, Swedberg K, Cleland JG, Di Lenarda A, Hanrath P, Komajda M, Lubsen J, Lutiger B, Metra M, Remme WJ, Torp-Pedersen C, Scherhag A, Skene A; Carvedilol Or MetoprololEuropean Trial Investigators. Comparison of carvedilol and

metoprolol on clinical outcomes in patients with chronic heart failure in the Carvedilol Or Metoprolol European Trial (COMET): randomised controlled trial. *Lancet.* 2003;362(9377):7-13.

[30] de Peuter OR1, Souverein PC, Klungel OH, Büller HR, de Boer A, Kamphuisen PW. Non-selective vs. selective beta-blocker treatment and the risk of thrombo-embolic events in patients with heart failure. *Eur J Heart Fail.* 2011;13(2):220-6.

[31] Weir MA, Dixon SN, Fleet JL, Roberts MA, Hackam DG, Oliver MJ, Suri RS, Quinn RR, Ozair S, Beyea MM, Kitchlu A, Garg AX. β-Blocker Dialyzability and Mortality in Older Patients Receiving Hemodialysis. *J Am Soc Nephrol.* 2014 Oct 30. pii: ASN.2014040324. [Epub ahead of print]

[32] Beta-blocker Heart Attack Trial Research Group: A randomized trial of propranolol in patients with acute myocardial infarction. I.Mortality results. *JAMA.* 1982;247(12):1707-14.

[33] Furberg CH, Hawkins M, Lichstein E, for the Beta Blocker Heart Attack Trial Study Group: Effect of propranolol in postinfarction patients with mechanical or electrical complications. *Circulation.* 1984;69(4):761-5.

[34] Maia ER, Villacorta H, Subietta CG, Munhoz C, Romêo Filho LJ, Mesquita ET. Use of propranolol in heart failure patients: safety, tolerability, and effects on left ventricular function. *Rev Port Cardiol.* 2001;20(4):383-99.

[35] Talwar KK, Bhargava B, Upasani PT, Verma S, Kamlakar T, Chopra P. Hemodynamic predictors of early intolerance and long-term effects of propranolol in dilated cardiomyopathy. *J Card Fail.* 1996;2(4):273-7.

[36] Greenblatt DJ, Koch-Weser J. Adverse reactions of propranolol in hospitalised medical patients: a report from the Boston Collaborative Drug Surveillance Program. *Am Heart J.* 1973;86(4):478-84.

[37] Authors/Task Force members, Elliott PM, Anastasakis A, Borger MA, Borggrefe M, Cecchi F, Charron P, Hagege AA, Lafont A, Limongelli G, Mahrholdt H, McKenna WJ, Mogensen J, Nihoyannopoulos P, Nistri S, Pieper PG, Pieske B, Rapezzi C, Rutten FH, Tillmanns C, Watkins H; Authors/Task Force members. 2014 ESC Guidelines on diagnosis and management of hypertrophic cardiomyopathy: the Task Force for the Diagnosis and Management of Hypertrophic Cardiomyopathy of the European Society of Cardiology (ESC). *Eur Heart J.* 2014;35(39):2733-79.

[38] Swanton RH, Brooksby IA, Jenkins BS, Webb-Peploe MM. Hemodynamic studies of beta blockade in hypertrophic obstructive cardiomyopathy. *Eur J Cardiol.* 1977;5(4):327-41.

[39] Speiser KW, Krayenbuehl HP. Reappraisal of the effect of acute betablockade on left ventricular filling dynamics in hypertrophic obstructive cardiomyopathy. *Eur Heart J.* 1981;2(1):21-9.

[40] Udelson JE, Cannon RO III, Bacharach SL, Rumble TF, Bonow RO. Beta-adrenergic stimulation with isoproterenol enhances left ventricular diastolic performance in hypertrophic cardiomyopathy despite potentiation of myocardial ischemia: comparison to rapid atrial pacing. *Circulation.* 1989;79(2):371-82.

[41] Bratt EL, Ostman-Smith I. Effects of lifestyle changes and high-dose β-blocker therapy on exercise capacity in children, adolescents, and young adults with hypertrophic cardiomyopathy. *Cardiol Young.* 2014:1-10. [Epub ahead of print]

[42] Hess OM, Grimm J, Krayenbuehl HP. Diastolic function in hypertrophic cardiomyopathy: effects of propranolol and verapamil on diastolic stiffness. *Eur Heart J.* 1983;4(suppl F):47-56.

[43] Hubner PJ, Ziady GM, Lane GK, Hardarson T, Scales B, Oakley CM, Goodwin JF. Double-blind trial of propranolol and practolol in hypertrophic cardiomyopathy. *Br Heart J.* 1973;35(11):1116-23.

[44] Flamm MD, Harrison DC, Hancock EW. Muscular subaortic stenosis. Prevention of outflow obstruction with propranolol. *Circulation.* 1968;38(5):846-58.

[45] Adelman AG, Shah PM, Gramiak R, Wigle ED. Long-term propranolol therapy in muscular subaortic stenosis. *Br Heart J.* 1970;32(6):804-11.

[46] Stenson RE, Flamm MD Jr., Harrison DC, Hancock EW. Hypertrophic subaortic stenosis. Clinical and hemodynamic effects of long-term propranolol therapy. *Am J Cardiol.* 1973;31(6):763-73.

[47] Frank MJ, Abdulla AM, Canedo MI, Saylors RE. Long-term medical management of hypertrophic obstructive cardiomyopathy. *Am J Cardiol.* 1978;42(6):993-1001.

[48] Sato H, Tateishi H, Uchida T, et al. Takotsubo type cardiomyopathy due to multivessel spasm. In: *Clinical aspect of myocardial injury: from ischemia to heart failure;* Kodama K, Haze K, Hon M, editors. Kagaku Hyoronsha; Tokyo, Japan: 1990. pp. 56-64.

[49] Sachdeva J, Dai W, Kloner RA. Functional and histological assessment of an experimental model of Takotsubo's cardiomyopathy. J Am Heart Assoc. 2014;3(3):e000921.

[50] Yoshioka T, Hashimoto A, Tsuchihashi K, Nagao K, Kyuma M, Ooiwa H, Nozawa A, Shimoshige S, Eguchi M, Wakabayashi T, Yuda S, Hase M, Nakata T,Shimamoto K. Clinical implications of midventricular obstruction and intravenous propranolol use in transient left ventricular apical ballooning (Tako-tsubo cardiomyopathy). *Am Heart J.* 2008;155(3):526.e1-7.

In: Propranolol
Editor: Mislav Puljević

ISBN: 978-1-63482-974-8

Chapter 5

Propranolol Use in Hyperthyroidism

Maja Baretić, MD PhD*
Internal Clinic, Department of Endocrinology,
University Hospital Centre Zagreb

Abstract

Hyperthyroidism is the principal endocrine indication for propranolol treatment. High levels of thyroid hormones result in a hyperdynamic cardiovascular state including increased stroke volume, augmented myocardial contractility and growth of the left ventricle. Thyroid hormones have a direct effect on the cardiovascular system. They increase cardiac output and lower systemic vascular resistance; also amplify intrinsic activity of sinoatrial node. Such actions lead to increased heart rate with a higher chance of supraventricular tachyarrhythmia, and the most common of them is atrial fibrillation. Thyroid hormones have positive chronotropic and dromotropic activity. Hyperthyroidism creates higher sensitivity to sympathetic stimulation which is conducted through greater number of β-adrenergic receptors. Myocytes contain an enzyme called type 2 deiodinase which increases local conversion T4 to T3. As a non-selective inhibitor of β-adrenergic receptors, propranolol is ideal for treating hyperthyroidism. By blocking β 1 receptors affects the sinoatrial and AV nodes propranolol lowers heart frequency, weakens myocardial contractions and leads to lower oxygen demand. By influencing β 2 receptors peripheral vasoconstriction rises. Thyroid hormone impact on β 2 receptors changes the activity of the peripheral 5'-monodeiodinase which converts T4 on the periphery in the active forms of T3. By using propranolol the tremor is reduced. Since the drug is lipophilic it crosses the bloodbrain barrier influencing central nervous system. With propranolol in hyperthyroidism there is less emotional lability and mental tension. The amount of the drug is 10-40 mg divided into 3-4 doses a day, and maximal dosage is 160 mg.

* Corresponding Address: KBC Zagreb, Zavod za endokrinologiju, Kišpatićeva 12, 10 000 Zagreb, Croatia; Mail maja.simek@zg.t-com.hr; Mobile 00385 98 41 2284; Fax 00385 2376036.

Introduction

Propranolol has, contrary to many other beta blockers, found its place in treating many diseases that are not related to the field of cardiology. Propranolol is used in treating migraines and anxiety. It is mentioned in treating refractory schizophrenia, essential tremor, infantile haemangioma, burns and oesophageal varices in liver cirrhosis. Beta blockers are rarely used in treating endocrinological diseases. Patients with elements of metabolic syndrome (obesity, hypertension, diabetes/glucose intolerance, dyslipidaemia) are rarely treated with that type of drugs because of their side effects, i.e., it is given only in cases when there is an inevitable cardiological indication. With diabetic patients beta blockers can overshadow the first warning signs of hypoglycaemia, with people having erectile dysfunction they can worsen the symptoms, and the treatment with patients having peripheral diabetic antipathy is questionable. Without the doubt, there are differences within the group of beta blockers for all of the above. The exception for using beta blockers in field of endocrinology is hyperthyroidism, the state in which the use of beta blockers is obligatory, and the one that stands out amongst them is propranolol.

Thyroid - Structure and Function

The thyroid is an endocrine gland located in the lower third of the neck, right below the cricoid cartilage. It has a butterfly like shape and consists of a left and right lobe and isthmus. It weighs about 20 grams. The thyroid is surrounded by a thin capsule, its connective tissue fits closely to the trachea. The main unit of its structure is a follicle. Follicle is surrounded by epithelial cells and filled with colloid. Epithelial cells which surround the follicle are thyrocytes - cubic cells responsible for the synthesis of thyroid hormones. Between the follicles there are C cells that secret calcitonin. Thyrocytes are typical glandular cells that secrete proteins; they are extremely metabolically active. Their endoplasmic reticulum and Golgi apparatus produce and secrete thyroglobulin. Thyroglobulin is big glycoprotein molecule secreted into the follicles. Thyrocytes have an apical side (near the colloid) and a basal side (near the membrane). The synthesis of thyroid hormones takes place under the influence of TSH (thyroid stimulating hormone) which is synthesized in the anterior pituitary. [1] TSH is a glycated protein which is made of non-covalently connected α and β subunits. The synthesis of TSH is regulated by a classic negative feedback loop in which the thyroid hormones directly inhibit the synthesis of TSH in the pituitary gland and indirectly regulate on the hypothalamus level where they decrease the secretion of TRH (thyrotropin-releasing hormone). [2] The synthesis of thyroid hormones is a complex process mainly performed in the thyroid gland, partly finished in the extrathyroidal tissues. Iodine is an essential trace element that enters into the composition of thyroid hormone. An adequate intake of iodine is required for the normal production of thyroid hormones. Iodine is imported in thyrocyte with the help of Na+/I- symporter (transmembrane protein). The process is stimulated with the help of TSH which activates receptors on thyrocyte basal membrane. TSH stimulation results with intracellular activation of adenylate cyclase through Gα-protein and the synthesized cyclic AMP (adenosine monophosphate). Result of TSH stimulation is increase of Na+/I- symporter synthesis. [3] After the iodine enters thyrocytes it transforms from non-organic form into organically bound iodine. First step is the oxidation of iodine with the help of enzyme TPO (thyroid peroxidase). It is followed by embedding of iodine and coalescing with thyroglobulin. In that way active thyroid hormones, T4 (thyroxin) and T3 (triiodothyronin), are formed. Synthesized thyroid hormones have to detach from thyroglobulin to get secreted. Microvilli on the apical side of the thyrocyte are formed under the influence of TSH and thyroglobulin is imported from the follicle lumen into thyrocyte. Thyroglobulin connects with lysosome which leads to its proteolysis. After the proteolysis of thyroglobulin, thyroxin is partly secreted and partly transformed into triiodothyronin in the process of deiodination. Deiodinase is an enzyme which takes part in the activation and deactivation of thyroid hormones. [4] T4 converts into T3 in the deiodinase process in thyroid gland, but also in the target cells of different tissues. There are several subtypes of deiodinases. Thyroid hormones are transmitted through blood by protein carriers, the most important of which is TBG (thyroxine–binding globulin) which carries 2/3 of bound hormones. A small part of the overall T3 and T4 are free in serum (not bound to carriers) and only the free hormones have effect on the target tissues. T3 and T4 fulfil their biological roles by binding to the receptor located in nucleus of the target cell. The receptors have a high affinity for triiodothyronin so most of the overall quantity of thyroid hormones bound to the receptors is T3. The receptors are located on the special part of the DNA (deoxyribonucleic acid). The hormones produce heterodimers with the receptor for retinoid X (RXR). By binding the thyroid hormones, the core's receptors are activated and they start the process of transcription and translation so the mRNA (messenger ribonucleic acid) is created. [5] The genetic influence of the thyroid hormones develops because of the increased activity of proteins created with the activation of intracellular receptors. However, thyroid hormones also have non-genetic influence through regulation of ion channels and oxidative phosphorylation through cAMP (cyclic adenosine monophosphate) or signal transduction of the kinase protein. Non-genetic influence of thyroid hormones can be seen on organs such as heart and pituitary gland, or fat tissue. [6] Thyroid hormones increase the number and membrane surface of the mitochondria in all the cells which directly influences metabolism. They increase the energy consumption with the activity of Na+/K+-ATPase pump. They influence the growth of children and brain development in foetus. The effect of the thyroid hormones on metabolism results in higher carbohydrate metabolism, faster entry of glucoses in the cells, faster glycolysis, gluconeogenesis, increased insulin production, and better absorption of carbohydrates. [7] Thyroid hormones speed up fat metabolism, decrease fat storage by mobilizing lipids, increase the concentration of fatty acids in plasma and their oxidation, but also lower cholesterol, phospholipids, and triglycerides in plasma. The effect of thyroid hormones on the respiratory system are an increase of the frequency and depth of breathing because of the higher consumption of O_2 and production of CO_2; it leads to increased bowel movement in the gastrointestinal tract and higher secretion of digestive enzymes; they influence the nervous system by speeding up the mental functions; they affect the power and contraction of muscles because of the increased stimulation of synapses in the parts of spinal cord that are in charge of muscle tone; they increase bone metabolism and blood flow through skin so the skin is warm and moist. Thyroid hormones have a special effect on the circulatory system. T3 and T4 enlarge the flow and cardiac output by speeding up the metabolism and consuming more oxygen which leads to vasodilatation. Higher heart frequency is caused by increased cardiac output or direct effect of hormones on the heart. It causes increased strength of heart contractions due to the higher enzymatic activity. Faster pulse follows the increased blood flow. Systolic pressure rises and diastolic pressure drops so the average arterial pressure stays the same. [8] When higher quantities of hormone are secreted, the basal metabolic rate can expand 60-100% above normal and all of the stated effects are increased. It is also important in the regulation of basal metabolic rate, so the change of its function leads to variations in body mass. Thyroid also influences an array of physiological processes which are all influenced by changes in hormone level. This gland is an organ that is highly dependent on immune changes and autoimmune diseases in the areas of adequate iodine saturation are its most common pathology.

Hyperthyroidism

Thyrotoxicosis is the state of higher level of free thyroid hormones in the serum followed by hypermetabolism. Hyperthyroidism is the state of increased thyroid activity and thyrotoxicosis is a broader term. Hyperthyroidism is classified as primary hyperthyroidism in which the thyroid secretes too much hormone and secondary one in which the pituitary gland stimulates the thyroid by the central action. The suppression of TSH is characteristic for primary hyperthyroidism and iatrogenic hyperthyroidism. Secondary hyperthyroidism, which is a rare disease, is followed by high or normal levels of TSH with higher thyroid hormones. Hyperthyroidism can develop at any age, although it is most common in females aged 20-50. It is 3-4 times rarer in males. The thyroid is a gland that regulates an array of metabolic processes in the organism so even the less prominent disorders of its function can produced a variety of clinical presentations in different age groups. Metabolic effects of the thyroid on the organism are the same in all forms of thyrotoxicosis and their intensity depends on age, general state of the organism, comorbidities, duration of the illness and the level of thyroid hormones. [9]

The clinical picture varies from mild subclinical chronic changes to acute state with severe manifestations. The clinical finding seen in the thyroid exam during hyperthyroidism can be normal, or the thyroid can be diffusely enlarged or there can be palpable nodes on the neck. During subacute thyroiditis the gland is very painful while palpating. Sometimes, due to increased flow through the thyroid, a so called Lian's murmur can be heard with a stethoscope.

The symptoms of hyperthyroidism related to increased level of hormones result in enhanced adrenergic tone. Patients complain of augmented mental tension, restlessness, emotional lability and insomnia. Mental changes occurring in thyroid gland dysfunction vary from mild mood swings to acute psychotic conditions. Older patients can also have an atypical picture with symptoms that are more similar to depression or dementia but without other manifestations of disease. Weight loss in spite of healthy or increased appetite is common. Weight loss varies from one case to another. Some patients do not lose weight at all, other lose up to 20 kg. Alongside faster metabolism, bowel movement is more frequent which explains frequent stools and additional weight loss. The skin is warm and moist, muscular weakness is present to the level of fasciculation, beside general weariness and fatigue. Thyrotoxic myopathy develops as a chronic toxic myopathy and is characterized by proximal muscle weakness. Acute myopathy, periodical paralysis, ophthalmoparesis, and neuromuscular transmission disturbances are less commonly seen. Postural tremor is typical for hyperthyreosis, it occurs when the patient maintains a position of arms against gravity, such as holding the arms outstretched. Tremor is most commonly discrete, but sometimes a more serious tremor can occur with prominent neurological symptomatology. A common occurrence is sweating, not being able to stand heat commonly mistaken for perimenopausal symptoms. Sometimes oligomenorrhea occurs (total absence of menstrual cycle is rare). Tachycardia, disturbances in heart rhythm (e.g., atrial fibrillation and heart failure, which is described separately) occur along with hyperthyroidism. [10] Cardiac pathology, especially arrhythmia, is common in older people with hyperthyroidism. The occurrence of angina pectoris and myocardial infarction are not rare in people with pre-existing changes in blood vessels. Thyrotoxic crisis is an acute life-threatening condition marked by a sudden occurrence of serious symptoms of hyperthyroidism alongside amplified body temperature, extreme anxiety and weariness, and it can lead to cardiovascular collapse. Thyroid storm is caused by untreated or maltreated hyperthyroidism but it can also be caused by an infection, a surgical procedure, pregnancy, or sudden suspension of thyrostatic drugs etc.

The most common cause of hyperthyroidism (70-80% of patients) is autoimmune thyroid disease (Morbus Graves or Basedow). [11] Autoimmune hyperthyroidism morphologically presents with evenly, diffusely changed thyroid. Hyperthyroidism is consequence of autoimmune event in which the antibodies for TSH receptor are produces. TSH receptor is glycoprotein with 764 amino acids; it is an thyroid specific antigen. The antibodies for that receptor imitate the function of TSH, they cause the stimulation of the gland. There are TSI and TSAb (thyroid stimulating immunoglobulin, thyroid stimulating antibodies). Antibodies that stimulate thyroid are not routinely measured. Autoimmune hyperthyroidism is a systemic disease with antibodies to attacking other organ with organ specific antigens like ones for oculomotor muscles and orbital fibroblasts. The consequence is ophthalmopathy responsible for exophthalmus. It is not necessary that ophthalmopathy follows the course of thyroid disease, it can occur with hyperthyroidism, but sometimes it even occurs earlier or later; sometimes just followed by the presence of antibodies in euthyreosis. The symptoms of orbitopathy are, alongside exophthalmus, changes on eyelids followed by widening of eyelid slit, retraction (lift eyelid like when you raise your eyebrows in wonder), eyelid oedema and protrusion of the bulbus. Patient can have diplopia or have inflammation of conjunctive or eyelids. Both eyes do not have to be affected equally. Pretibial oedema may also occur. More often other autoimmune diseases occur such as type 1 diabetes, vitiligo, pernicious anaemia, collagenosis, polyglandular syndrome, etc.

Toxic solitary thyroid nodule and multinodular goitre are the second most common cause of hyperthyroidism. Aetiology is probably a combination of multiple causes, dominantly mutation of genes for TSH receptor with permanent stimulation, but without autoimmunity. [12] The thyroid follicles become autonomous in creating thyroid hormones in nodes that are metabolically dominant. There are areas of abnormal growth in the thyroid that are not liable to mechanisms that normally control the thyroid. Those areas (or one area) produce thyroid hormones in large quantities. If there is one node that autonomously secretes thyroid hormones and suppress the surrounding tissue it is called a toxic adenoma. In toxic multinodular goitre and toxic adenoma there are no changes on the eyes. The symptoms are similar to the symptoms of Graves' disease but a little bit less prominent.

Inflammatory thyroid disease (subacute thyroiditis) is a type of thyrotoxicosis which occurs when, most probably, viral inflammation destroys the thyroid and the stored hormones are released. Symptoms of inflammation, fever, and severe neck pain occur. When the thyroid is inflamed like that, thyroid hormones are released due to the destruction of the gland, but condition later it often ends as hypothyroidism. [13]

Autoimmune thyroid inflammation is histologically seen as lymphocyte infiltration of thyrocytes and is, in honour of the author who first described it, called Morbus Hashimoto. That type of autoimmune thyroiditis can have multiple clinical forms: hypothyroidism, euthyroid state, hyperthyroidism, painless thyroiditis or postpartum thyroiditis. [14] Autoantibodies are directed towards thyroglobulin, the kD 670 protein which is synthesised in thyrocytes. TPO, known as a microsomal antigen, is the second most important antigen for the clinical practice. The immune disorder in Hashimoto thyroiditis is followed by the production of antibodies which lead to destroying the follicle epistle, immune inflammation, cytokines release which leads to destroying of the tissue. The dominant manifestation is hypothyroidism, but sometime hyperthyroidism occurs as a first symptom of destroying of tissue. A rare form of thyrotoxicosis is the initial state of increased secretion of beta HCG (human chorionic gonadotropin) a part of whose structure is similar to TSH (found in uterine choriocarcinoma, mollar disease, struma ovarii etc.). [15] One of the forms of thyrotoxicosis and iatrogenic intake of thyroid hormones is the so-called iatrogenic thyrotoxicosis (overdosing with medications that cure hypothyroidism). Some of the medication not related to treatment of thyroid disease can cause hyperthyroidism (lithium, interferon α or substances that contain iodine). A demanding issue is the treatment of hyperthyreosis caused by the amiodarone, an antiarrhythmic agent producing either hypothyreoidism or hyperthyroidism. Amiodarone is a medicine that has different levels of antiarrhythmic action, it prolongs phase 3 of the cardiac action potential, but the influence one thyroid is due to its iodine content. A 200 mg amiodarone pill contains 75 mg of iodine. The excess of T3 and T4 induced by amiodarone can be of hyperthyroidism type (increased stimulation of the thyroid) but also of thyrotoxicosis type (destroying of the thyroid by thyroiditis and secretion of hormones). The sole therapy depends on the subtype of hyperthyroidism induced by amiodarone; it is cured by thyrostatics and/or corticosteroids. Sometimes the difference is not entirely clear.

Secondary hyperthyroidism is caused by the pituitary gland tumour secreting TSH. That type of tumour secretes from pituitary thyrotrophic cells whole TSH molecule or α-/ β-subunit. The tumour does not respond to the suppression of thyroid hormones. These tumours are extremely rare and are discovered in an advanced stage. Usually thy are macroadenomas, larger than 10 mm. Together with hyperthyreosis, there are symptoms of local invasion of central nervous system (compressive symptoms with visual impairment, headaches, cranial nerve paralysis), or consequences of hypopituitarism (lower level of other pituitary gland hormones). [16]

Heart in hyperthyroidism

Hyperthyroidism leads to a hyperdynamic cardiovascular state followed by higher stroke volume and decreased peripheral vascular resistance. During the course of hyperthyroidism the effects of T3 and T4 on the heart are increased, the transport of adenosine into myocardial cells is higher, and the phosphorylation of adenosine is augmented. The excess of thyroid hormones changes the membrane ATPase (activated with potassium and sodium) and ATPase located in sarcoplasmic reticulum (activated with calcium). They both affect hearth muscle contraction. There is a possibility that their effect on the heart is a consequence of additional genetic activity through increased synthesis of α myosin and decreased activity of beta β myosin. The change of the α/β ratio is associated to increased myocardial contractility. As a consequence of the things stated above, during hyperthyroidism significant changes in contractility of the heart occur, followed with increased mass of the left ventricle. T3 has a direct effect on the heart which results in higher cardiac output and lower systemic vascular resistance. Sinoatrial node has increased intrinsic activity. It also leads to faster heart rate with a higher chance of supraventricular tachyarrhythmia and premature ventricular contractions. Clinically, the most common symptoms are palpitations and arrhythmia Thyroid hormones have positive, chronotropic and dromotropic effect. [17] The most common arrhythmia is atrial fibrillation. Even subclinical hyperthyroidisms greatly augment the risk of developing atrial fibrillation so TSH should be a routine check in every person with that type of disturbances in heart rhythm. Tachycardia developed in hyperthyroidism is resistant to digoxin. Cardioversion is advised if fibrillation is persistent and after 6 months of achieved euthyroidism. Along with atrial fibrillation thromboembolic incidents often occur, especially cerebrovascular ones. [18] Cardiac failure occurs more often in patients with pre-existing heart disease, more often in older patients. There are cases of cardiac failure during severe hyperthyroidism even without pre-existing heart weaknesses. Stroke volume is augmented, peripheral vascular resistance is lower, systolic blood pressure is increased, and diastolic lowered. The volume of plasma is increased with dilation of surface blood vessels producing skin changes. Sometimes a systolic murmur can be heard, a result of mitral valve prolapse in thyrotoxicosis. It is proved by echosonography and is reversible after the treatment, caused by insufficient delivery of ATPase in papillary muscle which has a shortened contraction time. Means-Lerman phenomenon is a murmur heard in the middle of systole above the upper left corner of sternum as a result of pericardia touching pleura in patient with hyperthyroidism. A similar murmur is heard in pericarditis. Patients with a pre-existing chronic heart condition often develop problems with angina, but they can also occur in people with normal coronary blood vessels because the myocardia's need for oxygen is increased. A chest x ray can vary from normal to cardiomegaly with decompensation; electrocardiogram shows increased voltage and a different disturbance in heart rhythm followed by prolonged PR interval. Increased beta adrenergic activity of the heart is also present. It occurs when thyroid hormones influence the heart muscle in genetic or non-genetic manner. Even a long-term subclinical hyperthyroidism influences the heart muscle. The consequence is diastolic dysfunction too. If it is a long-term process the changes are not reversible. Sympathomimetic activity and the activity of thyroid hormones lead to similar heart activity, especially when it comes to the strength and speed of heart muscle contraction. The state of hyperthyroidism leads to increased sensitivity to sympathetic stimulation. It was noticed that during the state of hyperthyroidism the level of catecholamine in plasma and urine is normal/lower which means that lower sympathetic stimulation leads to more intense response. [19] Increased activity of sympathicus is carried out through higher number of β adrenergic receptors. It was proved that thyroid hormones increase the number of β adrenergic receptors and Gs protein. There is evidence that there is presence of an enzyme called type 2 deiodinase in myocyte that augments the local conversion of T4 into T3, which is an active form. The heart muscle has both, β1 and β2 subtype of adrenergic receptors. β1 receptors make up 70% of all adrenergic receptors. The number of β adrenergic receptors is about two times higher in sinoatrial node than in other myocardial of tissue, and there are around 75% of β1 receptors for which T3 is responsible. β2 receptors are mostly located in the vascular structures of the heart. Under the influence of T3 mRNA synthetises multiple times more β1 adrenergic receptors, while the one for β2 receptors does not change significantly. Hyperthyroidism causes increased morbidity and mortality rates related to circulatory system. [20] Alongside curing hyperthyroidism, it is necessary to treat cardiac problems and its consequences on the circulatory system. It was proved that poor response to initial therapy (thyrostatics and radioactive iodine) is a bad prognostic sign. The opposite disease, hypothyroidism, also has negative effects on the heart and it is necessary to treat it by adding levothyroxine. In patients with pre-existing heart diseases that type of therapy should be introduced very carefully and gradually since exogenous T4 can lead to hyperthyroidism too. In older patients without pre-existing heart diseases immediate application of full dose of synthetic thyroid hormones can lead to the exposure of until then unknown heart disease. Patients with a history of heart disease or patients that might have a higher risk of heart disease should start with smaller doses, and the dose is gradually increased every week (severe cases of hypothyroidism and myxoedema are an exception).

Treatment of hyperthyroidism

There are several ways of treating hyperthyroidism. One of them is thyreostatic drug therapy with medicaments like propylthiouracil or thiamazole. Those drugs inhibit the synthesis of thyroid hormone by blocking the activity of TPO, i.e. by disabling the incorporation of iodine into organic compounds. They do not influence existing thyroid hormones deposited into the thyroid (i.e., thyroglobulin) or those that are present in circulation. They are administered perorally, first in higher doses and then the dose is gradually tapered. They are the first choice for people that do not have extremely high hormone levels and have a high chance of going into remission. Thyreostatic drugs are also the first choice for people that cannot be treated surgically and/or with radioiodine therapy due to some condition. If the doctors decide to treat the patient with medications only, it is necessary to continue the treatment even after achieved euthyroidism. The treatment should last at least 1-1.5 year because the thyreostatic drugs have an immunomodulatory effect, and too short use of those medications increases the probability of relapse of the disease. Potentially most serious side effect of thyrostaic drugs is agranulocytosis. There is possibility of the inhibition of the remaining myelopoietic cells (thrombocytopenia, aplastic anaemia). [21] Other side effects are hepatitis, drug fever, lupus-like syndrome, periarthritis and hypoprothrombinemia. [22] In the first trimester of pregnancy propylthiouracil therapy is the first choice, in other cases it is. Long-term treatment with thyrostatics (more than 2 years) is not the option, and if relapse occurs other choices of therapy should be explored.

Another option of treatment is application of radioactive iodine isotope. I-131 is built up in the thyroid tissue. The effect of the treatment is due to the tissue damage caused by radiation. Radioactive iodine treatment is administered in diffuse hyperthyroidism, multinodular goitre and toxic adenoma. The optimal dose of radiopharmaceutical is calculated prior to the administration of radioactive iodine. The mentioned dose is based on the absorbed radioiodine dose in thyroid tissue. Different countries (and institutions) position that type of therapy in different ways. Sometimes it is the first choice and sometimes it is administered as a second line (e.g., no possibility to cure the disease with medications, or in cases when it is not possible to control the increased level of hormone with drugs). It is also administered in cases when treatment with thyrostatic drugs had severe side effects, or with people that have previously undergone surgical procedure. Absolute contraindications for I-131 treatment are pregnancy and breastfeeding (i.e., when pregnancy is being planned). Relative contraindication is a more serious form eye-related symptom to, i.e., exophthalmus in autoimmune hyperthyroidism. Before radioiodine treatment thyroid cancer should be excluded too. The I-131 treatment is especially suitable for patients that cannot be surgically treated due to poor general condition and for older patients. Seeing that iodine 131 therapy often has delayed effect thyrostatic drug therapy can be administered for some time too (especially if hyperthyroidism is still present). It is also possible to additionally administer radioactive iodine treatment later. Treatment complications are rare. Most common is radiation-induced thyroiditis, i.e., sensitivity or pain in the thyroid and temporary increase of thyroid hormone level in blood 3-14 days after treatment. [23]

Surgical treatment is the first choice in cases when there is a suspicion of thyroid neoplasm or if there is a goitre causing compressive symptoms due to its volume and it cannot be expected that other treatments will lead to its significant downsizing. A relative indication is hyperthyroidism at a young age (although some countries prefer I- 131 as a first line of treatment), relapse after other forms of treatment and pregnancy planned in next 4-6 months. It is important for patient to be in euthyreosis (induced by thyrostatics and iodine solutions) before surgery. It is also necessary to improve the general state of a patient including stabilization of the heart rhythm. [24] It is still an open issue whether it is necessary to do a total thyroidectomy (removing the entirety of thyroid tissue) or partial thyroidectomy (removing the smaller part of the thyroid). Complications are damaging the laryngeal nerve and dysphonia. Sometime parathyroid glands are removed, and iatrogenic hyperparathyroidism occurs followed by and hypocalcaemia. All the side effects of general anaesthesia, not related to the thyroid gland may occur too.

Thyrotoxic crisis, without an option of waiting for the effects of iodine or medications, can also be treated surgically with prior medical treatment.

Alongside primary ways of treating hyperthyroidism, sedatives and other cardiovascular drugs are often administered, like diuretics, antihypertensive, in atrial fibrillation in higher doses of digoxin, anticoagulants etc.

Conclusion-Propranolol in Hyperthyroidism

Beta blockers are a group of drugs that antagonistically influence the β adrenergic receptors. They are distinguished by whether they predominantly block β 1 receptors (located in the heart muscle) or β 2 receptors (located in the smooth muscle tissue of bronchi and blood vessels) or both of them. If they block both groups of the receptors they are called non-selective beta blockers. Propranolol is one of the oldest non-selective inhibitor of beta adrenergic receptors. With the development of pharmacology many selective beta blockers were discovered that mostly influence β 1 receptors of the heart, used to achieve cardioselectivity. Those cardioselective beta blockers have in many conditions precedence over non-selective beta blockers because they avoid the effects on β 2 receptors. They ensure less bronchospasm, vasoconstrictions, and less prolonged hypoglycaemia in persons with diabetes. Cardioselectivity is relative term: when such drugs are administered in high doses, the influence on both types of receptors is expected.

Propranolol lowers heart frequency and weakens the contractions of the heart muscle by blocking β 1 receptors, also influencing sinoatrial and AV nodes. It also leads to lower oxygen demand in the heart which is beneficial effect in hyperthyroidism. Typical condition in hyperthyroidism is lower vascular resistance resulting in decreased stroke volume and sometimes leading to circulatory collapse and shock. By influencing β 2 receptors propranolol produces vasoconstriction and corrects the initially disorder caused by hyperthyroidism. Also, by influencing the β 2 receptors it changes the activity of peripheral 5'-monodeiodinase which converts T4 in active forms of T3 on the periphery. [25] Propranolol, unlike some other beta blockers, does not have intrinsic sympathomimetic activity and does not worsen the symptoms of hyperthyroidism. Propranolol therapy results with fewer tremor. As the medicine is lipophilic and crosses the blood–brain barrier, there is less emotional lability, mental tension but also less muscular weakness. If the patient has an obstructive pulmonary disease, Reynaud's phenomenon or some other contraindication, a selective beta blocker therapy can be given, or alternatively a non-dihydropyridine Ca-channel blocker like verapamil or diltiazem. [26] The amount of propranolol is divided into 3-4 doses per day and they can be 10 to 40 mg each. Total dose of propranolol varies. Some patients will require very high dose of 160 mg twice daily. Those are usually young patients in a very bad clinical condition. [27] When the patient is entering euthyreosis the dose of propranolol has to be appropriately lowered. Sometimes only small doses of medicine are prescribed with a possibility that the patient takes more drugs on demand (if they experience symptoms like tachycardia). Following propranolol therapy, as well as with the therapy of other beta blockers, the number of beta receptors is increased. Sudden suspension in beta blockers therapy can cause the so-called "rebound effect", a new and more powerful stimulus which has clinical symptoms the same as a hyperthyroidism relapse. Propranolol dose should be tapered gradually, taking into consideration thyroid home status.

FPP (familial periodic paralysis) syndrome is a rare autoimmune dominant disease with episodes of flaccid paralysis occurring with the loss of deep reflexes, without muscular response to electric stimulation. It is a genetic disease, the mutation of 1 q chromosome (HypoPP type I) is identified. There are four subtypes of this disease: hyperkalemic, hypokalemic, Andersen-Tawil syndrome and thyrotoxic. In the thyrotoxic type, episodes of paralysis last hours to days and are usually precipitated by exercise, stress, or a carbohydrate load. Symptoms of thyrotoxicosis are present usually months or years before paralysis, rear at the same time as periodic paralysis. Combined with other therapy, propranolol is mandatory used. [28]

In the other form of periodic paralysis called TPP (thyrotoxic periodic paralysis) in hyperthyroidism muscular paralysis occurs followed by hypokalaemia too. Genetic mutations in the L-type calcium channel α1-subunit ($Ca_v1.1$) have been described; the mutations are located in a different part of the gene from previously mentioned one in FPP. The background is an alteration of Na+/K+-ATPase on cellular membrane which becomes exposed due to hyperadrenergic stimulation during hyperthyroidism. In such cases propranolol has emergent indication. Beside curing hyperthyroidism and recovering potassium levels, the propranolol use is initial therapy.

References

[1] Dumont JE, Lamy F, Roger PP et.al. Physiological and pathological regulation of thyroid cell proliferation and differentiation by thyrotropin and other factors. *Physiological Rev.* 1992;72:667-97.

[2] Dumont JE. The action of thyrotropin on thyroid metabolism. *Vitam. Horm.* 1971;29:287-412.

[3] Dohan O, De la Vieja A, Paroder V et al. The sodium/iodide Symporter (NIS): characterization, regulation, and medical significance. *Endocr. Rev.* 2003;. 24:48-77.

[4] Bianco AC, Kim BW. Deiodinases: implications of the local control of thyroid hormone action. *J. Clin. Invest.* 2006;116:2571-9.

[5] Gurr JA, Kourides IA. Regulation of thyrotropin biosynthesis. Discordant effect of thyroid hormone on alpha and beta subunit mRNA levels. J Biol Chem. 1983;258:10208-11.

[6] Davis PJ, Davis FB, Cody V. Membrane receptors mediating thyroid hormone action. *Trends Endocrinol. Metab.* 2005;16:429-35.

[7] Freinkel N. Aspects of the endocrine regulation of lipid metabolism. In: Dawson MC, Rhodes DN, editors. Metabolism and physiological significance of lipids. New York: John Wiley & Sons Inc, 1965: 455.

[8] Woeber KA. Thyrotoxicosis and the heart. *N. Engl. J. Med.* 1992;327:94-98.

[9] Bahn Chair RS, Burch HB, Cooper DS et al. Hyperthyroidism and other causes of thyrotoxicosis: management guidelines of the American Thyroid Association and American Association of Clinical Endocrinologists. *Thyroid.* 2011;21:593-646.

[10] Frost L, Vestergaard P, Mosekilde L. Hyperthyroidism and risk of atrial fibrillation or flutter: a population-based study. *Arch. Intern. Med.* 2004;164:1675-8.

[11] Goldsmith RE. Radioisotope therapy for Graves' disease. *Mayo Clin. Proc.* 1972;47:953-61.

[12] Gabriel EM, Bergert ER, Grant CS et. al. Germline polymorphism of codon 727 of human thyroid-stimulating hormone receptor is associated with toxic multinodular goiter. *J. Clin. Endocrinol. Metab.* 1999;84:3328-35.

[13] Volpe, R. The management of subacute (DeQuervain's) thyroiditis. *Thyroid* 1993;3:253-55.

[14] Baretić M. 100 years of Hashimoto thyroiditis, still an intriguing disease. *Acta Med. Croatica*. 2011;65:453-7.

[15] Nagataki S, Mizuno M, Sakamoto S et.al. Thyroid function in molar pregnancy. *J. Clin. Endocrinol. Metab*. 1977;44: 254-63.

[16] McDermott MT, Ridgway EC. Central hyperthyroidism. *Endocrinol. Meta.b Clin. North Am.* 1998;27:187-203.

[17] Woeber KA. Thyrotoxicosis and the heart. *N. Engl. J. Med.* 1992;327:94-8.

[18] Sgarbi JA, Villaca FG, Garbeline B et.al. The effects of early antithyroid therapy for endogenous subclinical hyperthyroidism in clinical and heart abnormalities. *J. Clin. Endocrinol. Metab.* 2003; 88:1672-77.

[19] Tse J, Wrenn RW, Kuo JF. Thyroxine-induced changes in characteristics and activities of beta-adrenergic receptors and adenosine 3′,5′-monophosphate and guanosine 3′,5′-

monophosphate systems in the heart may be related to reputed catecholamine supersensitivity in hyperthyroidism. *Endocrinology*. 1980;107:6-16.

[20] Heeringa J, Hoogendoorn EH, van der Deure WM et al. High-normal thyroid function and risk of atrial fibrillation: the Rotterdam study. *Arch. Intern. Med.* 2008;168:2219-4.

[21] Amrhein JA, Kenny F, Ross D. Granulocytopenia, lupus-like syndrome, and other complications of propylthiouracil therapy. *J. Pediatr.* 1970;76:54-63.

[22] Baretić M, Balić S, Gudelj G. Myasthenic crisis as a side effect of methimazole therapy: case report. *Acta Clin. Croat*. 2010;49:67-71.

[23] Sisson JC, Freitas J, McDougall IR et al. Radiation safety in the treatment of patients with thyroid diseases by radioiodine ^{131}i: practice recommendations of the american thyroid association. *Thyroid.* 2011;21:335-46.

[24] Feely J, Crooks J, Forrest AL et.al. Propranolol in the surgical treatment *Br. J. Surg.* 1981;68:865-9.

[25] Wiener L, Stout BD, Cox JW: Influence of beta sympathetic blockade with propranolol on the hemodynamics of hyperthyroidism. *Am. J. Med.* 46:227, 1969.

[26] Dahl P, Danzi S, Klein I. Thyrotoxic cardiac disease. Curr. Heart Fail. Rep. 2008;5:170-6.

[27] ACC/AHA/ESC Practice Guidelines ACC/AHA/ESC 2006 Guidelines for the Management of Patients with Atrial Fibrillation. A*m. Coll. Cardiol*. 2013;61(18):1935-44.

[28] Shah M, Mutneja R, Vyas Det.al. Thyrotoxic hypokalemic periodic paralysis: two case reports and a brief review of literature. *Conn. Med.* 2013;77:487-9.

In: Propranolol
Editor: Mislav Puljević

ISBN: 978-1-63482-974-8

Chapter 6

Propranolol Use in Patients with Liver Cirrhosis

***Irena Hrstić*[1,*] *and Rajko Ostojić*[2]**
[1]Pula General Hospital, School of Medicine, University of Zagreb, Zagreb, Croatia
[2]University Hospital Zagreb, School of Medicine, University of Zagreb, Zagreb, Croatia

Abstract

Approximately half of patients with cirrhosis have esophageal varices. One-third of all patients with varices will develop variceal hemorrhage, a major cause of morbidity and mortality among patients with cirrhosis. Pre-primary prophylaxis refers to measures aimed at preventing the development of varices. Primary prophylaxis aims to prevent variceal hemorrhage in patients with esophageal varices who do not have a history of hemorrhage, whereas secondary prophylaxis aims to prevent hemorrhage in patients with a history of variceal hemorrhage. An ideal treatment of portal hypertension would be one that is universally effective, safe, easy to administer and cost-effective.

Nonselective beta-adrenergic blockers reduce portal pressure by reducing portal venous inflow as a result of a decrease in cardiac output and splanchnic blood flow. Several studies have proved that nonselective beta-blockers prevent variceal hemorrhage in patients with varices.

1. Introduction

Liver cirrhosis is defined histologically as a diffuse hepatic process characterized by fibrosis and the conversion of normal liver architecture into structurally abnormal nodules. Liver injury may develop into cirrhosis over weeks to years. Liver cirrhosis presents the end stage of any progressive chronic liver disease. Regardless of the uniformity of the term "end stage", liver cirrhosis is usually divided into three phases according to the Child-Pugh

* Corresponding author: Ass. Prof. Irena Hrstić, MD, PhD, Pula General Hospital Aldo Negri 6, 52100 Pula, Croatia, E-mail: irena.hrstic@gmail.com.

classification. In each phase, the possibility of survival and the occurrence of complications differ.

The Child-Pugh score was originally developed in 1973 to predict surgical outcomes in patients with bleeding esophageal varices. **[1]** Since then, it has been modified and become a widely used tool to assess prognosis in patients with chronic liver disease and cirrhosis. The score considers five factors. Three factors assess the synthetic function of the liver (total bilirubin, serum albumin and international normalized ratio) and the remaining two are based on clinical assessment (degree of ascites and degree of hepatic encephalopathy), see Table 1.

Having in mind that liver cirrhosis is the end stage of any untreated chronic liver disease and that several factors (viral, metabolic, toxic, autoimmune and genetic) can cause chronic liver disease, liver cirrhosis is a major health problem. Untreated liver cirrhosis will undoubtedly result in functional deterioration (decompensation) and/or malignant transformation and, finally, death. Clinical signs of liver cirrhosis are treatable, and if the underlying cause is not curable, at this stage, liver cirrhosis can at least be stabilized.

The leading causes of cirrhosis in the Western world are alcohol and hepatitis C, however, the occurrence of non-alcoholic liver disease (NAFLD) has been considerably rising. NAFLD is one of the features of the metabolic syndrome which also includes hypertension, dysregulated glucose homeostasis, dyslipidemia, obesity and others. Consequently, an increasing numbers of patients with chronic liver disease or liver cirrhosis are on antihypertensives for essential hypertension. For years, beta-blockers have been considered the basis for the treatment of hypertension as well as a good treatment for the prevention of hemorrhage from varices in patients with liver cirrhosis.

Portal hypertension is one of the clinical syndromes that present liver cirrhosis. At the phase of portal hypertension, the chronic liver disease underlying cirrhosis has reached the end stage when the chronicity is irreversible.

2. Portal Hypertension

Portal hypertension is a frequent clinical syndrome. Normally, vascular channels of the liver are smooth and portal vein pressure ranges between 1–4 mm Hg higher than the hepatic vein free pressure, and not more than 6 mm Hg higher than right atrial pressure. At the stage of liver cirrhosis with scarring, the liver parenchyma vascular channels become irregular and tortuous with accompanying increased resistance to flow. This increases the pressure gradient between the portal vein and the inferior vena cava above normal levels, and when the portal pressure gradient rises above 10 mmHg, portal hypertension becomes clinically significant and complications of portal hypertension usually arise. Clinical signs of developed portal hypertension are formation of ascites, encephalopathy and formation of gastroesophageal varices.

2.1. Natural History of Varices

Gastroesophageal collaterals and varices develop from connections between the short gastric and coronary veins and the esophageal, azygos and intercostal veins. In advanced cirrhosis, over 80% of portal blood may circulate through these collaterals. Collateral resistance will have a marked influence on portal pressure.

The presence of gastroesophageal varices correlates with the severity of liver disease. Gastroesophageal varices are present in approximately half of patients with compensated cirrhosis, 60% of those with ascites and eventually almost all of the patients will have them. Varices develop at a rate of 7% to 8% per year and the transition from small to large varices occurs at the same rate. [2] Consequently, the general consensus is that endoscopy should be repeated after 2–3 years in patients without varices on initial endoscopy. Patients with HVPG ≥10 mmHg have two- to three-fold risk of developing varices and these patients should have repeat endoscopy every 1–2 years. [3] Based on an expected 10–15% yearly rate of progression of variceal size, endoscopy should be repeated every year in patients with small varices to detect the progression from small to large varices.

2.2. Complications of Varices

Variceal hemorrhage occurs at a rate of 5% to 15% per year depending on the presence of risk factors. Patients at higher risk for variceal hemorrhage are those with large varices (15% per year), those with red wale marks on variceal wall and with liver cirrhosis in Child B or C stage. [4] Bleeding from varices stops spontaneously in up to 40% of patients, and regardless of therapy improvements, the six-week mortality with each episode of hemorrhage is at least 20% and it also depends on the severity of liver disease. [5] Patients with the hepatic venous pressure gradient (HVPG) >20 mmHg compared to those with lower pressure are at a higher risk for early rebleeding (within the first week); have less chance to control the bleeding (83% vs. 29%) and have a higher 1-year mortality (64% vs. 20%). [6] Late rebleeding occurs in approximately 60% to 70% of untreated patients, usually within 1 to 2 years of the initial hemorrhage. [7]

3. Nonselective Beta Blockers as Pharmacological Therapy for Portal Hypertension

Pharmacological therapy consists of splanchnic vasoconstrictors (vasopressin with analogues, somatostatin and analogues and nonselective-blockers) and venodilators (nitrates). Vasoconstrictors mainly act by producing splanchnic vasoconstriction and reducing portal venous inflow.

Propranolol and nadolol are nonselective beta blockers (NSBBs). Both of them reduce portal blood flow and, consequently, portal pressure by means of two mechanisms: by decreasing cardiac output (beta-1 effect) and inducing splanchnic vasoconstriction (beta-2 effect). NSBBs are one of the most effective preventative therapies in patients with cirrhosis against variceal bleeding. [8]

It has been well known for more than three decades that propranolol has a significant role in reducing the risk of rebleeding from esophageal varices. The first trial (RCT) took place in France in 1981, when Lebrec and colleagues showed on 74 patients with cirrhosis and a history of gastrointestinal bleeding that propranolol is superior than placebo in preventing variceal rebleeding (96% vs. 50%). [9]

Pre-primary prophylaxis aims to prevent the development of esophageal varices and some experimental studies have suggested that NSBBs can have a role in preventing the development of collateral circulation. [10, 11] Unfortunately, only few studies have been performed to test this hypothesis in humans and failed to prove the thesis. The results of a large multicenter placebo controlled study on 213 patients with cirrhosis without varices and HVPG >6 mmHg showed that NSBBs did not prevent the formation of varices and were even associated with an increased number of adverse events requiring discontinuation of treatment. [12] In patients with early cirrhosis, the ineffectiveness of the NSBB therapy can be attributed to a milder splanchnic and systemic hyperdynamic circulatory state. As a result, the use of NSBBs in pre-primary prophylaxis of variceal bleeding is currently not indicated. [13]

On the other hand, several studies have attempted to show on what size of varices NSBBs will have an effect in terms of decreasing the size and the rate of increasing in size. Cales and colleagues reported on 206 cirrhotic patients with small or no varices that an increase in size of varices over a period of one year was more frequent in patients treated with NSBBs, as compared to those on placebo. [14] On the other hand, Merkel and co-workers showed a trend towards a decreased progression of varices (from small to large) in patients treated with nadolol as compared to placebo. [15]

The challenges and adverse effects of NSBBs seem to be most obvious in patients with advanced cirrhosis and refractory ascites. Once again, in a different study a few decades after the first NSBB study, Lebrec and colleagues showed that the use of NSBBs in patients with decompensated cirrhosis may be associated with poor survival rates. [16] In their prospective observational study, 151 cirrhotic patients with refractory ascites regularly underwent large-volume paracentesis with concomitant intravenous albumin administration. They were divided into subgroups according to administration of NSBBs. The median survival rate was radically lower in patients treated with propranolol (5 vs. 20 months) with 19% probability of survival at 1 year, compared to 64% probability in no NSBB group. They further concluded that NSBBs are associated with the development of paracentesis-induced circulatory dysfunction.

Table 1. Child-Pugh classification of the severity of cirrhosis

	1 point	2 points	3 points
Encephalopathy	None	Grade 1-2 (or suppressed with medication)	Grade 3-4 (or refractory)
Ascites	None	Mild-Moderate	Severe
Bilirubin (mg/dL or μmol/L)	<2 or <34	2-3 or 34-45	>3 or >50
Albumin (g/dL)	>3.5	2.8-3.5	<2.8
INR	<1.7	1.71-2.30	>2.30
Severity according to the score	Class A total score 5-6	Class B total score 7-9	Class C total score ≥10
1-year survival	100%	80%	45%

3.1. Dosing of NSBBs

Although the recommended dosing of propranolol for the treatment of arterial hypertension in patients who are not cirrhotic is 4 times a day, in cirrhosis, twice a day dosing is sufficient because of a slower drug metabolism. The starting dosage is 20 to 40 mg orally twice a day and this is gradually increased to a maximum of 160 mg twice a day.

The dose of NSBBs can be titrated by measuring patient's heart rate or by measuring hepatic venous pressure gradient. The latter is not used in daily practice, because it is not widely available as well as due to its invasiveness. However, a very convenient method is to adjust the dose according to baseline resting heart rate.

In many randomized controlled trials the dose was adjusted to obtain a 25% decrease in heart rate; however, recent guidelines have recommended the adjustment of NSBBs to the highest tolerated dose or to a heart rate of 50 to 55 beats/min. [17]

If the heart rate remains elevated despite maximal doses of NSBBs, the first thing that should be taken into account is patient compliance. If the patient is adherent to medication, propranolol can be used intravenously followed by the measurement of hepatic venous pressure gradient. This method can differentiate the patients who are unlikely to respond to NSBBs from those who need higher dose or will probably adhere poorly to medication. In good responders, hepatic venous pressure gradient will drop immediately by 10% to 20% or will be <12 mmHg.

Conclusion

For more than 3 decades, the use of propranolol has proven to be satisfactorily safe in patients with liver cirrhosis and developed portal hypertension with varices. Several studies have proven that propranolol plays a significant role in preventive therapy, especially in patients with small varices that have not bled but have criteria for increased risk of hemorrhage. Furthermore, it can be used in patients with medium or large varices that have not bled but meet criteria for bleeding. Few recent studies have advised caution with regard to patients with refractory ascites, but the data is inconsistent and further investigation is required.

References

[1] Pugh, RN; Murray-Lyon, IM; Dawson, JL; Pietroni, MC; Williams, R. Transection of the oesophagus for bleeding oesophageal varices. *Br J Surg.*, 1973, 60(8), 646-649.

[2] Merli, M; Nicolini, G; Angeloni, S; Rinaldi, V; De Santis, A; Merkel, C; Attili, AF; Riggio, O. Incidence and natural history of small esophageal varices in cirrhotic patients. *J Hepatol.*, 2003, 38(3), 266-272.

[3] Bosch, J; Abraldes, JG; Berzigotti, A; García-Pagan, JC. The clinical use of HVPG measurements in chronic liver disease. *Nat Rev GastroenterolHepatol.*, 2009, 6(10), 573-582.

[4] North Italian Endoscopic Club for the Study and Treatment of Esophageal Varices. Prediction of the first variceal hemorrhage in patients with cirrhosis of the liver and esophageal varices. A prospective multicenter study. *N Engl J Med*, 1988, 319, 983-989.

[5] Carbonell, N; Pauwels, A; Serfaty, L; Fourdan, O; Lévy, VG; Poupon, R. Improved survival after variceal bleeding in patients with cirrhosis over the past two decades. *Hepatology*., 2004, 40(3), 652-659.

[6] Moitinho, E; Escorsell, A; Bandi, JC; Salmerón, JM; García-Pagán, JC; Rodés, J; Bosch, J. Prognostic value of early measurements of portal pressure in acute variceal bleeding. *Gastroenterology*., 1999 Sep, 117(3), 626-631.

[7] Bosch, J; García-Pagán, JC. Prevention of variceal rebleeding. *Lancet*., 200315, 361(9361), 952-954.

[8] Mehta, G; Abraldes, G; Bosch, J. Developments and controversies in the managements of esophageal and gastric varices. *Gut*, 2010, 59, 701-705.

[9] Lebrec, D; Poynard, T; Hillon, P; Benhamou, JP. Propranolol for prevention of recurrent gastrointestinal bleeding in patients with cirrhosis, a controlled study. *N Engl J Med*, 1981, 305, 1371-1374.

[10] Lin, HC; Soubrane, O; Cailmail, S; Lebrec, D. Early chronic administration of propranolol reduces the severity of portal hypertension and portal-systemic shunts in conscious portal vein stenosed rats. *J Hepatol*., 1991, 13, 213-219.

[11] Sarin, SK; Groszmann, RJ; Mosca, PG; et al. Propranolol ameliorates the development of portal-systemic shunting in a chronic murine schistosomiasis model of portal hypertension. *J Clin Invest*., 1991, 87, 1032-1036.

[12] Groszmann, RJ; Garcia-Tsao, G; Bosch, J; et al. Beta-blockers to prevent gastroesophageal varices in patients with cirrhosis. *N Engl J Med*., 2005, 353, 2254-2261.

[13] De Franchis R. Revising consensus in portal hypertension: report of the Baveno V consensus workshop on methodology of diagnosis and therapy in portal hypertension. *J Hepatol*., 2010, 53, 762-768.

[14] Calés, P; Oberti, F; Payen, JL; et al. Lack of effect of propranolol in the prevention of large oesophageal varices in patients with cirrhosis: a randomized trial. French-Speaking Club for the Study of Portal Hypertension. *Eur J GastroenterolHepatol*., 1999, 11, 741-745.

[15] Merkel, C; Marin, R; Angeli, P; et al. A placebo-controlled clinical trial of nadolol in the prophylaxis of growth of small esophageal varices in cirrhosis. *Gastroenterology*., 2004, 127, 476-484.

[16] Serstè, T; Melot, C; Francoz, C; Durand, F; Rautou, PE; Valla, D; Moreau, R; Lebrec, D. Deleterious effects of beta-blockers on survival in patients with cirrhosis and refractory ascites. *Hepatology*., 2010 Sep, 52(3), 1017-22.

[17] Garcia-Tsao, G; Sanyal, AJ; Grace, ND; et al. Prevention and management of gastroesophageal varices and variceal hemorrhage in cirrhosis. *Hepatology*, 2007, 46, 922-938.

In: Propranolol
Editor: Mislav Puljević

ISBN: 978-1-63482-974-8

Chapter 7

Propranolol Use in Psychiatry

Martina Bojanić, MD, and Vesna Barić, MD
University Psychiatric Hospital Vrapče, Zagreb, Croatia

Abstract

INTRODUCTION: In the sympathetic nervous system, there are three subtypes of beta-adrenergic receptors (adrenoceptors) called beta 1, beta 2 and beta 3. They are distributed throughout different body areas. Beta 1 and beta 2 receptors are found in the brain. Beta blockers represent a widely used group of drugs in clinical practice. In this chapter, we will describe one of the most commonly used beta-blockers that is called propranolol. Propranolol is the non-selective antagonist of beta 1 and beta 2 adrenergic receptors and possesses some antagonist activity at the serotonin 5-HT1A receptors. In general, all beta blockers reach the central nervous system, but the more lipid soluble beta blocker penetrates the central nervous system (CNS) more extensively.

INDICATION IN PSYCHIATRIC DISORDERS: Propranolol can be used as an adjunctive treatment for panic disorder (PD), when patients have failed to respond to several standard treatments. However, the real effectiveness of propranolol in this indication remains unclear and need to be further investigated. It is mostly reserved for patients who have failed to respond to several first-line treatments. Treatment recommendations for general anxiety disorder are very similar to panic disorder, but the adjuvant treatment with propranolol did not show significant efficacy. Propranolol is widely used for the treatment of social phobia, primarily of the performance type. In the literature, data can be found about the effectiveness of propranolol use in posttraumatic stress disorder (PTSD). Propranolol showed promise in blocking memory consolidation and reconsolidation in healthy individuals. Future studies are trying to investigate whether they can also be weakened in patients with posttraumatic stress or other event-related disorders. The use of propranolol can be beneficial for medication-induced postural tremors, especially for lithium-induced postural tremor. Many studies suggest that beta blockers are effective for the treatment of aggressive and violent behaviors, especially those related to organic brain syndrome. Propranolol can be beneficial in patients with mild to moderate withdrawal, by reducing the autonomic nervous system manifestations of a withdrawal.

CONCLUSION: In general, beta blockers demonstrated effectiveness in various psychiatric disorders. They are definitely effective in social phobia, lithium-induced postural tremor, and neuroleptic-induced akathisia. They are probably effective as an adjunctive therapy for alcohol withdrawal and other substance-related disorders, as well as an adjunctive therapy for aggressive or violent behavior. Beta blockers are possibly effective in antipsychotic and antidepressant augmentation.

Sympathetic nervous system (which is part of autonomic nervous system) is playing very important role in many physiological functions in the body, e.g. increases arterial blood pressure and cardiac output, increases blood flow to the brain, heart and skeletal muscles, increases blood glucose and muscle strength, also increases sweating and rate and depth of respiration etc. The sympathetic nervous system is stimulated by physical or emotional stress that stimulates different protective mechanisms (above mentioned) designed to help the individual to cope with stress or get away from it [1]. The physiological responses resulting from activation of the sympathetic nervous system are mediated by noradrenaline (NA) and adrenaline (A). Both compounds activate specific membrane receptors called adrenoceptors. Medications called beta-adrenergic receptor antagonists (also known as beta-blockers) are preventing the binding of noradrenaline and adrenalin to beta-adrenoceptors.

In the sympathetic nervous system, there are three subtypes of beta-adrenergic receptors called beta 1 (β 1), beta 2 (β 2) and beta 3 (β 3). They are distributed throughout different body areas. Beta 1 and beta 2 receptors are found in the brain. Unfortunately, the adequate technique for visualization of beta adrenoreceptors in the human brain is not yet available. There were found two radioligands: *S*-1'-^{18}F-fluorocarazolol and *S*-1'-^{18}F-fluoroethylcarazolol (analogs of potent beta blocker carazolol), that could actually visualise receptors in human brain, but they were found to be mutagenic and cannot be used in human studies any more. Most of information that we have today are available from animal experiments, postmortem studies and very limited studies in humans. According to these observations, it is known that beta adrenoreceptors in the human brain are predominantly located in the cerebral cortex, nucleus accumbens and striatum. At lower densities, they are also located in amygdala, hippocampus and cerebellum [2, 3].

Beta blockers represent a widely used group of drugs in clinical practice. In this chapter, we will describe one of the most commonly used beta receptor antagonists, that is called propranolol. In general, propranolol is the non-selective (with equal affinity to both receptors) antagonist of beta 1 and beta 2 adrenoceptors and possesses some antagonist activity at the serotonin 5-HT1A receptors [4]. In general, all beta blockers reach the central nervous system, but the more lipid soluble beta blocker penetrates the central nervous system (CNS) more extensively.

Propranolol is highly lipophilic and, therefore, crosses the blood–brain barrier. According to FDA (Food and Drug Administration), propranolol is completely absorbed when taken per orally (only about 25% of propranolol reaches the systemic circulation), it crosses placenta and is distributed into breast milk. Approximately 90% of circulating propranolol is bound to plasma proteins. Propranolol is extensively metabolized by the liver. *In-vitro* studies have indicated that propranolol is catalyzed mainly by polymorphic CYP2D6. In healthy subjects, no difference was observed between CYP2D6 extensive metabolizers (EMs) and poor metabolizers (PMs). Propranolol can also inhibit the metabolism of diazepam, resulting in increased concentrations of diazepam and its metabolites. In contrary, diazepam does not alter the pharmacokinetics of propranolol. The pharmacokinetics of oxazepam, triazolam, lorazepam, and alprazolam are not affected by propranolol. Co-administration of chlorpromazine with propranolol resulted in a 70% increase in propranolol plasma level. The hypotensive effects of MAO inhibitors or tricyclic antidepressants (TCAs) may be exacerbated when administered with propranolol. Hypotension and cardiac arrest have been reported with the concomitant use of propranolol and haloperidol. It is known that propranolol is contraindicated for use in asthma, insulin-dependent diabetes, congestive heart failure, significant vascular disease, persistent angina, and hyperthyroidism. It can also worsen atrioventricular (AV) conduction defects. The most common side effects are hypotension and bradycardia, and in a risk group, a test dosage of 20 mg a day of propranolol should be given. In literature, depression as an adverse effect of beta blockade has been increasingly questioned, but, in fact, it is very rare. Central nervous system (CNS) adverse effects (e.g. agitation, confusion, and hallucinations) have also been reported and are very rare. However, it is important to emphasize that older patients may be at greater risk for neuropsychiatric side effects [5].

The Use of Propranolol in Psychiatric Disorders

In general, beta blockers (especially non-selective propranolol) demonstrated effectiveness in various psychiatric disorders. According to Kaplan and Sadock, they are definitely effective in social phobia (e.g. performance anxiety), lithium-induced postural tremor, and neuroleptic-induced akathisia [4]. They are probably effective as an adjunctive therapy for alcohol withdrawal and other substance-related disorders, as well as an adjunctive therapy for aggressive or violent behavior. Beta blockers are possibly effective in antipsychotic and antidepressant augmentation.

A number of case reports and controlled studies have proposed their role in many different areas of psychiatry that are very promising for the future. In this chapter, we will also present you some of them.

Anxiety Spectrum Disorders

It is important to observe anxiety within a complex biopsychosocial framework. The most important function of anxiety is preparing the individual both biologically and psychologically to meet various challenges and conflicts. Thus, symptoms of anxiety can be psychological, physical or a mixture of both. In general, anxiety is characterized by unreasonable feelings of fear, tension and panic that are very often associated with insomnia and impairment of concentration [6]. There are also physical disturbances-palpitations, tachycardia, tremulousness, sweating, diarrhea, etc. due to over-activity of the autonomic, particularly the sympathetic, nervous system. There are three major psycho-physiological aspects of anxiety: elevated sympathetic activity, autonomic inflexibility and asymmetrical patterns of brain activation [7].

The pharmacological treatments of anxiety spectrum disorders tend to be chronic, and are very complex. First line treatments include antidepressants: selective serotonin reuptake inhibitors (SSRIs) or selective serotonin and noradrenaline reuptake inhibitors (SNRIs), benzodiazepines (in more severe cases, often used as second-line options) and also psychotherapy. Tricyclic antidepressants (TCAs) are also effective but are less well tolerated than the SSRIs/SNRIs. Pharmacological treatment is indicated when symptoms become disabling or reduce the quality of life [8].

In the literature, a potential effect of propranolol on anxiety was mentioned for the first time in the 1966. when Granville-Grossman and Turner published article named: The effect of propranolol on anxiety [9]. They explained that beta blockers relieved manifestations of anxiety which are due to stimulation of peripheral beta receptors and that they inhibited the physiological response to emotional arousal. Thus, the authors propose the indication for their use in anxiety when the patient is troubled by prominent somatic symptoms, what is also proposed in later studies.

APA (American Psychiatric Association) guidelines emphasized that SSRIs, SNRIs, TCAs, and benzodiazepines have demonstrated their efficacy and are recommended for treatment of panic disorder [10]. Monoamine oxidase inhibitors (MAOI) also appear effective for panic disorder. Propranolol can be used as an adjunctive treatment for panic disorder (PD), when patients have failed to respond to several standard treatments. It is proposed that propranolol can be effective in panic disorder because it influences autonomic anxiety symptoms. However, the real effectiveness of propranolol in this indication remains unclear and need to be further investigated. It is mostly reserved for patients who have failed to respond to several first-line treatments.

Treatment recommendations for general anxiety disorder are very similar to panic disorder, but the adjuvant treatment with propranolol did not show significant efficacy.

Propranolol is widely used for the treatment of social phobia, primarily of the performance type (e.g. disabling anxiety before a musical performance or before public speaking). The usual dosage range is between 10 and 40 mg of propranolol, 20 to 30 minutes before the anxiety-provoking situation. When taking propranolol for the first time, it is proposed to take a "test dose" before, in order to be sure that the patient won't experience any adverse effects [4].

There is growing number of studies that are trying to explore how noradrenaline is involved in memory processing. In fact, the idea is that noradrenaline could be an important modulator of memory through its ability to activate both presynaptic and postsynaptic adrenergic receptors at central synapses with different functional outcomes. It is known that emotional arousal leads to activation of the locus coeruleus with the release of noradrenaline in the brain, resulting in the enhancement of memory. Also, authors are referring to the previous studies that provided evidence that emotional arousal facilitates memory consolidation, and that can be blocked by beta-blockers (e.g. propranolol) [11].

In the literature, data can be found about the effectiveness of propranolol use in posttraumatic stress disorder (PTSD). Growing number of studies have investigated the effect of propranolol on PTSD, consolidation and reconsolidation of emotional memories. That is according to data that during trauma exposure, endogenous stress hormones (i.e. noradrenaline) over consolidate the traumatic memory. PTSD and numerous psychiatric disorders actually have at their core a negative and sometimes traumatic emotional memory. Propranolol showed promise in blocking memory consolidation and reconsolidation in healthy individuals. Future studies are trying to investigate whether they can also be significantly weakened in patients with posttraumatic stress or other event-related disorders [12, 13].

Lithium-Induced Postural Tremor

The use of propranolol can be beneficial for medication-induced postural tremors, especially for lithium-induced postural tremor. Tremor occurs frequently as a side effect of lithium, a commonly used mood stabilizer. Lithium tremor is classified as a postural tremor and it can occur both at rest and while moving. In fact, lithium induces a fine postural tremor of the hands (frequency 8 to 12 Hz). Usually, the tremor does not affect patients' everyday activities, but an exacerbation of the tremor or its extension to other parts of the body may indicate rising lithium levels [14]. If possible, the initial approach should be lowering the lithium dose, eliminating aggravating factors (e.g. caffeine) and administering lithium at bedtime. According to Kaplan and Saddock, if these interventions are inadequate, propranolol can be effective in dose range 20 and 160 mg a day, given two or three times daily. Some authors proposed nadolol for lithium- induced tremor in the presence of liver damage [15].

Akathisia, Neuroleptic-Induced Acute Akathisia

The term drug-induced movement disorder (DIMD), represents a wide, treatment-emergent involuntary movements including akathisia, tardive dyskinesia, dystonia, and parkinsonism. Akathisia may be induced by various psychotropic agents, especially by first generation antipsychotics (conventional neuroleptics) and some atypical antipsychotics. Akathisia is an inner sensation of restlessness and an irresistible urge to move body parts. It is clinically presented as increased motor activity. Dysphoria is a major component of neuroleptic-induced akathisia and includes an inner sense of restlessness (often in the legs), anxiety and the urge to move. A common problem in everyday clinical practice is to distinguish akathisia from psychomotor agitation associated with the psychiatric disorder (especially the one associated with psychosis). Akathisia may also be a possible contributor to aggressive or suicidal behavior, and is crucial to be recognized and properly treated. Symptoms of acute akathisia may occur between one hour and several weeks after initiating or increasing the dose of medication. Management of neuroleptic-induced acute akathisia includes a dose reduction and switching to an atypical antipsychotic or alternative agent with less risk of akathisia. Administration of a lipophilic non-selective beta-blocker, such as propranolol can be effective. It seems that beta 2 receptor inhibition appears to be crucial for that efficacy. A dose range suggested as effective is between 30 mg and 90 mg of propranolol a day [16, 17].

Aggression and Violent Behavior

Many studies suggest that beta blockers are effective for the treatment of aggressive and violent behaviors, especially those related to organic brain syndrome. The major side effects of beta blockers, when used to treat aggression, are lowering of blood pressure and pulse rate. After brain injury, agitation and aggression are the most troublesome among all other psychiatric symptoms. The effectiveness of propranolol in reducing agitation and aggression in people who acquired injury has been reported. However, better evaluations are needed because it is difficult to distinguish additive from its independent effects [18].

For example, different psychotropic medications are frequently prescribed for neuropsychiatric symptoms (NPS) associated with dementia. In patients with Alzheimer's disease, there is enhanced behavioral responsiveness to central nervous system and noradrenaline (NE) that may contribute to the pathophysiology of disruptive behaviors such as aggression, uncooperativeness, irritability etc. It is important to emphasize that aggression in patients with Alzheimer's disease and other forms of dementia is very difficult to treat. The scientific evidence for safety and efficacy of beta-blockers in the treatment of aggressive behavior has never been definite. A placebo-controlled trial of the beta-blocker propranolol demonstrated improvement in NPS symptoms scores and global improvement in NPS [19]. Above mentioned placebo-controlled trial included thirty-one subjects (mean age, 85 ± SD 8) that were randomly assigned to take either propranolol or placebo for 6 weeks. Other psychotropic drugs were maintained constant. Authors concluded that short-term propranolol augmentation treatment (mean achieved dosage is 106 +/- 38 mg a day) appeared modestly effective and well tolerated for overall behavioral status in patients with probable or possible Alzheimer's disease complicated by disruptive behaviors. Propranolol may be helpful specifically for aggression and uncooperativeness. The propranolol treatment in this population was limited by the high frequency of relative contraindications to beta-adrenergic antagonist treatment.

Another example is the use of propranolol in the treatment of behavioral problems in adults with intellectual disability. People with intellectual disability often present behavioral problems, aggression is among the commonest. The management of aggression in that group is a clinical challenge and involves both behavioral management and medications. Sometimes, behavioral problems are triggered when patient with intellectual disability is situated in the unfamiliar environment and is frightened (e.g. during hospital admission). Behavioral management is very important and often forgotten, but in a very aggressive or uncooperative patient, pharmacotherapy may be required. There is a wide range of medications that can be used, such as lithium, anticonvulsants, and antipsychotics [20, 21]. Many authors indicate that propranolol may be effective in reducing aggression in a variety of neurologic and psychiatric conditions. It may also be effective in the self-injurious behavior commonly seen in the intellectually disabled. Therefore, low-dose propranolol may be a valuable treatment option in the management of aggression in intellectually disabled adults [21]. In general, beta blockers have demonstrated efficacy in moderate aggressive behavior, particularly explosive-aggressive episodes. Beta-blockers (especially lipophilic propranolol) in dose range between 80 to 280 mg a day per orally can cause short-term sedation and is less likely to cause long-term sedation induced by other medications [20]. For example, authors of a case report described a young man with a moderate intellectual disability and generalized epilepsy, who presented severe aggression. He was given a trial of propranolol, starting at 20 mg a day and increased by 20 mg every week. At 40 mg a day, there was a significant reduction in his aggression, and on further increasing the dose to 60 mg a day, aggression was completely reduced. Finally, he has been well on carbamazepine 1,000 mg a day, propranolol 60 mg a day, and diazepam 10 mg a day without episodes of seizures or aggression [21].

As mentioned before, beta-blockers showed efficacy in reducing aggression in a variety of neurologic and psychiatric conditions. We will describe one example from a literature that is both neurologic and psychiatric condition (agitation and aggression after severe traumatic brain injury). Severe traumatic brain injury (TBI), defined as a Glasgow Coma Scale ≤ 8, increases intracranial pressure and activates the sympathetic nervous system. Sympathetic hyperactivity manifests as an increase of noradrenaline and adrenaline levels, hypertension, abnormal heart rate variability and agitation. It is important to note that this is not unique to TBI and has also been observed after other intracranial processes. In a literature review, the authors of several articles have suggested that exposure to beta blockers may improve mortality rates following TBI [22]. It is presumed that the neuroprotective effects of beta blockers may be mediated by reducing cerebral metabolism and slowing of the catecholamine-induced catabolic state.

Alcohol Withdrawal

There are alcohol studies suggesting novel hypothesis that elevated noradrenergic signaling is an etiological factor in the abuse of a wide range of substances, including alcohol, nicotine, marijuana, heroin, cocaine, and caffeine. Also, they suggest that noradrenergic signaling is altered during acute intoxication, chronic use, acute withdrawal and stress-induced relapse or reinstatement of drug and alcohol use [23]. Therefore, propranolol can be beneficial in patients with mild to moderate withdrawal, by reducing the autonomic nervous system manifestations of a withdrawal. In general, beta-blockers inhibit the increased heart rate and control the tremor characteristic for hyperadrenergic states such as that of alcohol withdrawal. It is important to emphasize that propranolol does not have anticonvulsant activity and that effectiveness is not proved in reducing seizures or delirium [24]. Therefore, propranolol is useful as an adjuvant to benzodiazepines, but not as a single medication in the treatment. Suggested schedule for propranolol administration is: 50 mg propranolol for a pulse rate between 50 and 79 and 100 mg propranolol for a pulse rate of 80 or above [4]. When a pulse rate is below 50, no propranolol is given.

Autism

A group of authors presented the review of literature in order to find is there a role of a beta adrenergic blockade in autism spectrum disorder (ASD). They mentioned that until now, a significant association between beta-adrenoceptors and autism has been demonstrated. For example, some studies showed that plasma and urine NA levels were increased in ASD patients [25]. Also, in one study, propranolol (a 40 mg) attenuated cognitive impairment associated with ASD, which implicated that NA may play an important role in cognitive impairment (associated with ASD) [26]. There are also other theories of possible role of beta blockers in ASD e.g. via the suppression of MHC class II antigen expression, apoptotic factor or suppression of NAPDH expression, role in modulating the inflammatory processes. Some authors found high frequencies of the Gly16 and Glu27 alleles in the β-adrenergic receptor polymorphisms in patients with autism [27].

References

[1] K. M. Brophy, H. Scarlett-Ferguson, K. S. Webber, A.C. Abrams, C. Barnett Lammon. Clinical Drug Therapy for Canadian Practice, 2 ed. Philadelphia: Wolters Kluwer Health/Lippincott Williams & Wilkins; 2010.

[2] van Waarde A. and colleagues. Imaging Beta-Adrenoceptors in the Human Brain with (5)-l'-[18F] Fluorocarazolol. *J. Nucl. Med.* 1997 Jun; 38(6): 934-9.

[3] van Waarde A., Vaalburg W., Doze P., Bosker FJ, Elsinga PH.. PET imaging of beta-adrenoceptors in human brain: a realistic goal or a mirage?. *Curr. Pharm. De.* 2004; 10 (13): 1519-36.

[4] Sadock BJ, Sadock Alcott V. Kaplan and Sadock's synopsis of psychiatry, 10 ed. Philadelphia: LWW; 2007.

[5] T. Markham Brown, A. Stoudemire. Psychiatric Side Effects of Prescription and Over-The-counter Medications: Recognition and Management. Washington: *Amer. Psychiatric. Pub.* ; July 15, 1998.

[6] Granville-Grossman K. Propranolol, anxiety and the central nervous system. *Br. J. clin. Pharmac.* 1974; 1: 361-363.

[7] H. Barlow D. Anxiety and Its Disorders: the Nature and Treatment of Anxiety and Panic, 2 ed. New York: The Guilford Press; 2004.

[8] M. Stahl S. Stahl's essential psychopharmacology, 3 ed. New York: Cambridge University Press; 2008.

[9] Granville-Grossman KL, Turner P. The effect of propranolol on anxiety. *Lancet* 1966; 1: 788-790.

[10] Work Group on Panic Disorder. American Psychiatric Association (APA). Practice guideline for the treatment of patients with panic disorder. *Am. J. Psychiatry* 1998; 155(5): 1-34.

[11] PTSP Tully K, Y Bolshakov V. Emotional enhancement of memory: how norepinephrine enables synaptic plasticity. *Tully and Bolshakov Molecular Brain 2010*; 3: 15.

[12] Pitman RK, Orr SP. The black hole of trauma. *Biol. Psychiatry* 1990; 27: 469-71.

[13] Lonergan MH, Olivera-Figueroa LA, Pitman RK, Brunet A. Propranolol's effects on the consolidation and reconsolidation of long-term emotional memory in healthy participants: a meta-analysis.. *J. Psychiatry Neurosci.* 2013; 38(4): 222-31.

[14] J. Perry P. Psychotropic Drug Handbook, 8 ed. Baltimore: Lippincott Williams & Wilkins; 2007.

[15] Dave M, Langbart MM. Nadolol for lithium tremor in the presence of liver damage. *Ann. Clin. Psychiatry* 1994 ; 6(1): 51-2.

[16] American Psychiatric Association. Practice Guidelines for the Treatment of Psychiatric Disorders. Arlington: American Psychiatric Association; 2006.

[17] E. Tisdale J, A. Miller D. Drug-Induced Diseases: Prevention, Detection, and Management, 2 ed. Bethesda: ASHP; 2010.

[18] Fleminger S, Greenwood R, Oliver D. Pharmacological management for agitation and aggression in people with acquired brain injury. *Cochrane Database Syst. Rev.* 2006; (4): CD003299.

[19] Peskind E.R et colleagues. Propranolol for disruptive behaviors in nursing home residents with probable or possible Alzheimer disease: a placebo-controlled study. *Alzheimer Disease and Associated Disorders* 2005; 19: 23–28.

[20] Lindsay P. Care of the Adult with Intellectual Disability in Primary Care. London: Radcliffe Publishing Ltd; 2011.

[21] Rajkumar RP. Successful Management of Difficult-to-Treat Aggression With Low-Dose Propranolol in a Patient With Intellectual Disability: A Case Report. *Prim. Care Companion CNS Disord.* 2012; 14(5): PCC.12l01373.

[22] Tran TY, Dunne IE, German JW. Beta blockers exposure and traumatic brain injury: a literature review. *Neurosurg. Focus* 2008; 25(4): E8.

[23] J. Fitzgerald P. Elevated Norepinephrine may be a Unifying Etiological Factor in the Abuse of a Broad Range of Substances: Alcohol, Nicotine, Marijuana, Heroin, Cocaine, and Caffeine. *Subst. Abuse* 2013; 7: 171-183.

[24] K. Ries R, C. Miller S, A. Fiellin D. Principles of Addiction Medicine, 4 ed. Philadelphia: LWW; 2009.

[25] Barthelemy C et colleagues. Urinary free and conjugated catecholamines and metabolites in autistic children. *J. Autism Dev. Disord.* 1988; 18(4): 583-91.

[26] Narayanan A, White CA, Saklayen S, Scaduto MJ, Carpenter AL, Abduljalil A. Effect of propranolol on functional connectivity in autism spectrum disorder-a pilot study. *Brain Imaging Behav.* 2010; 4(2): 189-97.

[27] vinh quốc Lương K, Hoàng Nguyễn LT. The role of beta-adrenergic receptor blockers in autism. *American Journal of Psychiatry and Neuroscience* 2013; 1(1): 14-21.

In: Propranolol
Editor: Mislav Puljević

ISBN: 978-1-63482-974-8

Chapter 8

Propranolol Use in Neurology

Marina Puljević, MD
University Hospital Centre Zagreb,
Department of Neurology, Croatia

Abstract

Although propranolol is not cardioselective and has little intrinsic sympathomimetic activity, it has strong membrane stabilizing properties. This effect is mediated by the voltage gated sodium channels in cardiac, neuronal and skeletal tissues. It is also highly lipid soluble. About 2/3 of propranolol quality in the blood crosses the blood-brain barrier in a single passage. Although the cardiovascular system is considered as main target organ, propranolol has been also used in neurological disorders. Some of them are essential tremor, prophylaxis of migraine, postural tachycardia syndrome, sympathetic storming after severe traumatic brain injury and enhancement of antiepileptic drug potential. Essential tremor is one of the most common neurologic movement disorders often resulting in functional disability and leading to many physical and emotional difficulties. The 2005 American Academy of Neurology practice parameter gave a level A recommendation of efficacy to the β-adrenergic blocker propranolol and the anticonvulsant primidone. Another review reported convincing evidence only for propranolol. Propranolol is therefore only drug approved by the US Food and Drug Administration. Propranolol is also registered as Level A drug in prophylaxis of migraine according to the 2012 AHS/AAN Guidelines. Also, propranolol is found useful in postural tachycardia syndrome (POTS). Menagement of POTS is targeted at relieving low blood volume or regulating circulatory problems that could be causing the disorder, hence it includes avoidance of precipitating factors, volume expansion, physical countermaneuvers, exercise training, pharmacotherapy, pressure garments and behavioral-cognitive therapy. Numerous studies have also demonstrated anticonvulsant effects of antiarrhythmic drugs, moreover among beta-blockers (class II), propranolol showed anticonvulsant features in models for generalized tonic-clonic and complex partial seizures through direct membrane-stabilizing effects related to Na+ channel blockade, like some classical antiepileptic drugs. Due to the fact that propranolol suppresses sympathetic outflow, neuronal activity, decreases serum levels of catecholamines, reduces cardiac workload and inhibits central fevers by acting directly within the central nervous system it is also used in sympathetic storming after severe traumatic brain injury.

Introduction

Propranolol is a sympatholytic nonselective beta blocker. It blocks the epinephrine and norepinephrine action on both β1 and β2 adrenergic receptors. Due to inhibitory effects on norepinephrine transporter, propranolol also stimulates norepinephrine release in synapse, resulting with not only blocking β-adrenoreceptors, but also α-adrenergic activation. Therefore, it can be looked upon as an indirect α1 agonist and β antagonist. Although propranolol is not cardioselective and has little intrinsic sympathomimetic activity, it has strong membrane stabilizing properties through the ability to block cardiac, neuronal and skeletal voltage gated sodium channels and is highly lipid soluble.

As highly lipophilic drug it achieves high concentration in the brain, it crosses the blood-brain barrier and the placenta. About 2/3 of propranolol in the blood crosses the blood-brain barrier in a single passage, moreover propranolol injected into the carotid artery or intravenously is almost immediately present in the brain. Olesen et al. [1] studied regional cerebral blood flow with the ^{133}Xe-intraarterial injection method. Fifteen minutes after the propranolol infusion a normal reaction of CBF to changes in arterial $PaCO_2$ was found. Olesen had confirmed that propranolol infused locally was probably washed out and had been distributed to the whole body. As the result it was concluded that the 10 mg should be enough to ensure complete cardiovascular β-adrenergic blockade, but not enough to block parenchymal β-receptors in the brain.

Although the cardiovascular system is the main target organ, it has been also used in neurological disorders. Indications are: essential tremor, prophylaxis of migraine, postural tachycardia syndrome, sympathetic storming after severe traumatic brain injury, as well as improvement of antiepileptic drug potential.

Propranolol Use in Essential Tremor

Essential tremor (ET) is one of the most common neurologic movement disorders affecting 0.5% to 5% of the general population [2]. Its prevalence (0.9%) is comparable to that of epilepsy (0.7%), moreover tremor severity and handicap vary widely, and there are still most patients who did not receive a diagnosis and hence never treated. Although the prevalence of all ages is about 0.9%, for people aged 65 years and older it is 4.6% [3]. Essential tremor often results in functional disability, leading to many physical and emotional difficulties. ET is estimated to be a disease or family of diseases with aetiological, clinical and pathological heterogeneity. Epidemiological studies have identified several risk factors for ET: age, ethnicity, family history, environmental factors. Studies have shown an age-associated rise in the incidence and prevalence of ET. [4]

Genetic factors have been viewed as important in the aetiology of ET, linkage has been reported on gene ETM1 on chromosome 3q13 et ETM2 on chromosome 2p22-25 [5, 6], although it can occur sporadic also. According to two epidemiological studies [7, 8] implicated environmental factors are highly tremorogenic chemicals - β-carboline alkaloids (harmine, harmane) and lead. In terms of pathophysiology, clinical, physiological and imaging studies point to an involment of the cerebellum and/or cerebellothalamocortical circuits. Additionally, it was indicated that the majority of ET cases with changes in the cerebellum had Lewy bodies or neuronal depletion in the brainstem, mainly in the locus coeruleus [9, 10, 11].

Chung et al. in their study assessed the pattern of cortical thickness and diffusion tensor white matter changes in patients with ET according to the response to propranolol to explore the pathogenesis underlying the clinical heterogeneity of ET due to the fact that propranolol is one of the most widely used and efficacious antitremor drug, front-line agent. Imaging and clinical parameters were analyzed. Their data suggest that patients with ET have heterogeneous cortical thinning and white matter alteration with respect to responsiveness to propranolol, suggesting that its responsiveness may be a predictive factor to determine ET subtypes in terms of neuroanatomical heterogeneity [12].

Moreover, non-responders exhibited reduced cortical thickness, and the responders had greater disintegration of white matter. It is assumed that about 30% of patients with ET do not respond to propranolol, and some cases show tolerance to the drug effect with chronic treatment [13]. Mechanism of propranolol's antitremor effects has not been fully established. Some studies have suggested that it may act on peripheral beta-adrenoreceptors in the muscle fibers or spindles [14]and on the other hand some studies supported a possible role via a central action [15], through locus coeruleus as the primary source of noradrenergic innervations and due to the fact that it expresses beta-adreno receptors or through modulation of Renshaw cells, mediated indirectly via inputs from neurons expressing beta-adrenoreceptors, based on changes in corticomuscular coherence patterns according to Baker et al. [16]. However, considering pathogenesis of ET neurodegenerative changes are most pronounced in the cerebellum, impairment of Purkinje synapses is a component of cerebellar degradation that could underlie ET through the selective loss of Purkinje cells and signs of their axonal swelling as well as degeneration with formation of axonal torpedoes [9].

Therefore, any lesion in coerulo-cerebellar pathway may lead to alteration in the function of the Purkinje cells and disintegration of the cerebello–thalamo–cortical loop [17]. Furthermore, recent post mortem studies have evidenced alterations in LINGO 1 (leucine rich repeat and Ig domain containing 1) gene and GABA receptors in the cerebellum of people with ET. The diagnosis of ET remains exclusively clinical and several sets of diagnostic criteria have been proposed. The consensus criteria of the Movement Disorders Society's Tremor Investigation Group are probably most widely used. Occurrence of bilateral, largely symmetrical postural tremor with or without kinetic tremor affecting hands or forearms lasting for more than 5 years and presenting with a gradual onset is typically considered definite ET. Tremor may affect also other body segments, cranial musculature may be involved in 30% of cases, including neck-head or vocal cords, or occasionally the trunk, legs, feet, tongue and other facial musculature. Although, diagnostic criteria for definite ET require the presence of symmetrical postural and kinetic tremor, strictly unilateral kinetic tremor may be found in 10% to 20% of patients with presumed ET.

The frequency of the tremor is between 4 Hz and 12 Hz, and is inversely related to age, with older patients generally exhibiting tremor frequencies that are at the lower end of this range. It occurs only when the affected muscle is exerting effort, moreover any sort of physical or mental stress will tend to make the tremor worse. Tremorcan worsen also in response to fatigue, strong emotions, low blood sugar, cold and heat, caffeine, lithium salts, some antidepressants, and other factors. It is typical for the tremor to worsen in "performance" situations. ET is generally rhythmic tremor with a low amplitude in early stages, which increases with progression and high frequency. Kinetic tremor occurs during many voluntary movements, including writing, pouring, eating, and other daily activities, and it is the most recognized feature of ET. Patients with severe ET also have a postural tremor, which can be elicited by asking them to hold their arms outstretched in front of their bodies [18]. In general, the tremor is slowly progressive, but eventually producing disabilities with basic daily activities, severely affected end-stage patients are physically unable to feed or dress themselves. In these patients, the tremor prevents any normal activity, resulting in a substantial loss of independence and even incapacitation.

According to studies, 15–25% of clinic patients are forced to retire prematurely. It is well known its somatotopic spread over time, from the arms to the head. Head tremor typically develops several years after the onset of arm tremor, and the converse (spread of tremor from the head to the arms) is distinctly unusual. Some patients may have unsteadiness and problems with gait and balance, through several studies postural instability and ataxic gait in patients were noted. Also, some patients with ET develop tremor at rest [19].

Patients with rest tremor had disease of longer duration and of greater severity than those without rest tremor. Its therapy remains purely symptomatic, all medications used for the reduction of tremor have initially been developed and approved for other indications. Widespread pathological oscillation occurs throughout the motor system in patients with ET, and drugs presumably interfere with these oscillations. The 2005 American Academy of Neurology practice parameter [20] gave a level A recommendation of efficacy to the β-adrenergic blocker propranolol and the anticonvulsant primidone, whereas another review reported convincing evidence for efficacy of propranolol only [21].

The specific mechanism of propranolol's antitremor effects has not been fully established, although it is widely accepted that blocking effects of peripheral noncardiac β-2 receptors located in the muscle spindles are most likely responsible for the efficacy of propranolol in ET [22]. The effect of propranolol on tremor was first shown in 1965, and since then, several controlled trials have confirmed the efficacy of this medication in ET. Through trials it showed not only safety but also and efficacy, although efficacy is established only for tremor affecting the upper extremities, while head tremor response is quite limited. Propranolol is also beneficial in treatment of exaggerated physiological tremor that cannot be reliably distinguished from early stages of ET. The average tremor reduction was about 50% when compared with placebo, with highest percentage of 70%.Propranolol and primidone have been compared with one another in some studies.

According to Koller et al. in a study of 25 patients with ET, acuteadverse reactions occurred in 8% with propranolol and 32% with primidone,however, after 1 year significant side-effects occurred in 0% of patients treated with primidone compared with 17% taking propranolol. Although initial tolerability is a sizeable problem with primidone, long-term tolerability of primidone is superior to that of propranolol according to Koller et al. [23] However, only propranolol is approved by the US Food and Drug Administration. It is estimated that about 50% of patients have lasting benefit, with tolerance developing in about 14% and with assumption of about 30% of non responders to propranolol. Sustained release propranolol is as effective as conventional propranolol. Consequently, treatment should begin with initial dose of 30-60 mg per day, and the dose gradually increases, as needed, based on efficacy and tolerability.

Total daily dose of 60-320 mg per day is adequate in most patients. There is no convincing evidence that doses higher than 320 mg/day provide any additional benefit. Mentioned adverse effects are seen in up to 66% of treated patients, but they tend to be mostly mild. Dropout rates to significant side effect are estimated to be below 20%, and they are generally seen with daily doses more than 120 mg. The initiation dose in the geriatric population should be lower, 10 mg twice a day may be better tolerated in these patients. Even though only propranolol is supported by sufficient data to consider it as a first line therapy, other nonselective and selective β-blockers have been trialed in ET, and none of these is FDA approved for tremor control, only metoprolol and atenolol may be considered in patients who experience bronchospasm when treated with propranolol, but their tremor control tends to be much less robust and transient [24]. Primidone and propranolol may be used in combination when monotherapy is insufficient [20]. Second line therapy include gabapentin, pregabalin, topiramate, clonazepam, alprazolam, atenolol, metoprolol, and third line include nimodipine and clozapine. For patients with essential hand tremor that fails to respond to oral agents, botulinum toxin A is considered. It may also reduce head and voice tremor, but hoarseness and swallowing difficulties might occur after use for voice tremor [25]. Patients with refractory tremor may benefit from invasive therapies, such as deep brain stimulation and thalamotomy. The electrodes for deep brain stimulation are usually placed in the "tremor center" of the brain, the ventral intermediate nucleus (VIN) of the thalamus. Non-prescription agents such as ethanol have also traditionally played a part in the treatment of ET.

Propranolol Use in Migraine

Propranolol is also registered as Level A drug in prophylaxis of migraine according to the 2012 AHS/AAN Guidelines, together with divalproex sodium, sodium valproate, topiramate, metoprolol, timolol, petasites (butterbur) and frovatriptan for short-term prevention of menstrual migraine. Comparing AHS/AAN Guidelines with Canadian Guidelines and EFNS Guidelines it is notable that propranolol is placed in the highest tier along with divalproex, metoprolol and topiramate assigned to the top category in all 3 of the guidelines [26].

Migraine is a neurovascular disorder in a genetically predisposed individuals that affects approximately 12% of patients in the United States and millions worldwide. The exact mechanisms of migraine are not known. The primary theory is related to increased excitability of the cerebral cortex and abnormal control of pain neurons in the trigeminal nucleus of the brainstem. Diffuse projections from the locus caeruleus to the cerebral cortex result in impaired cerebral cortical blood flow causing the spreading depression associated with migranous auras (a transient visual, sensory, language, or motor disturbance which signals that the headache will soon occur). Typically the headache affects one half of the head, is pulsating in nature, and lasts from 2 to 72 hours. Associated symptoms may include nausea, vomiting, and sensitivity to light, sound, or smell. The pain is generally made worse by physical activity. It is a common, disabling, and costly disorder. There is no cure, but preventive treatment to decrease the number and severity of headache attacks improves health outcomes and quality of life as well as reduces disability and costs. Women are affected disproportionally, with a 3-fold higher prevalence which peaks between age 25 and 55 years, affecting the most productive years of a life [27]. More frequent and severe cases with significant impact on quality of life and daily activities may benefit from headache prophylaxis.

Despite reducing the frequency of migraine, the goal of prophylaxis is also to reduce painfulness and duration as well as to increase the effectiveness of abortive therapy. Another reason for prevention is to avoid medication overuse headache, in which the headaches become more severe and more frequent. It is a common problem and can result in chronic daily headache. This may occur with triptans, ergotamines, and analgesics, especially narcotic analgesic. [28] Prophylactic migraine therapy may be considered in these indications:

- frequency of migraine attacks is greater than 2 per month
- duration of individual attacks is longer than 24 hours
- the headaches cause major disruptions in the patient's lifestyle, with significant disability that lasts 3 or more days
- abortive therapy fails or is overused
- symptomatic medications are contraindicated or ineffective
- use of abortive medications more than twice a week and on time (within 15 minutes of pain onset)
- migraine variants such as hemiplegic migraine or rare headache attacks producing profound disruption or risk of permanent neurologic injury [29]

The decision to take preventative treatment is an individual one for the patient, however it should be considered when migraine frequency or severity increases to a point where it is interfering significantly with work, school, or social life. Although some patients see relief from prophylaxis, unfavorable side effects may limit tolerability and thus impact the effectiveness. The choice of treatment can be influenced to varying degrees by the particular pattern of migraine, patient co-morbidity, tolerability, teratogenecity, potential side effects, ease of use as well as patient choice. A study that explored the extent to which migraine patients are willing to tolerate side effects of prophylaxis found that the top reasons why a prophylactic is deemed intolerable to patients are weight gain (divalproex),cognitive effects like memory loss and depression (topiramate),somnolence(amitriptyline and propranolol).[30] There are three main aspects of treatment: trigger avoidance, acute symptomatic control, and pharmacological prevention. Preventative treatment should be commenced at a low dose, to minimise the possibility of developing side effects. Recommended dose for propranolol is 20-320 mg per day, it should be started at 20-30 mg daily (in divided doses) and increased steadily. However, during pregnancy prophylaxis with β-blockers because of the association with intrauterine growth retardation should be avoided, if necessary it should be used in lowest possible dose. Beta-blockers such as propranolol and metoprolol have been used as preventative treatments for migraine since the 1970s. They are effective treatments, especially for patients with frequent migraines interspersed by periods of headache freedom. Preventive migraine medications are considered effective if they reduce the frequency or severity of the migraine attacks by at least 50%. Silberstein et al. conducted a double-blind, placebo-controlled, randomized clinical trial to assess the efficacy and safety of adding propranolol to topiramate in chronic migraine [31]. The results from this study suggest that the combination of topiramate with propranolol does not provide clinically relevant benefit over topiramate alone in a chronic migraine population.

Propranolol Use in Postural Tachycardia Syndrome

Postural tachycardia syndrome (POTS) is a heterogeneous disorder defined by a heart rate increment of 30 beats/min or more within 10 minutes of standing or head-up tilt in the absence of orthostatic hypotension; the standing heart rate is often 120 beats/min or higher [32]. Although the underlying cause of POTS remains unclear, several mechanisms have been proposed including sympathetically mediated vasoconstriction, excessive sympathetic drive, hypovolemia and deconditioning. Several studies registered a decrease in systolic and diastolic cerebral blood flow velocity by 44% and 60% [33]. POTS manifests with symptoms of cerebral hypoperfusio (light-headedness, blurred vision, fainting, cognitive difficulties, and generalized weakness) and excessive sympathoexcitation (palpitations, chest pain, tremulousness).The faintness or lightheadedness of POTS are relieved by lying down again. It is more frequent in women (4.5:1), moreover, most cases occur between the ages of 15 and 25 years and often begins after a pregnancy, major surgery, trauma, or a viral illness. Physical deconditioning and psychological factors have an important role in these patients, indeed, endurance exercise training decreases standing heart rate, restores blood volume, and improves orthostatic tolerance and associated symptoms. The term orthostatic intolerance is used to describe a condition in which patients develop symptoms on standing or head-up tilt but do not fulfill the heart rate criteria for the diagnosis of POTS [34]. POTS has been classified into several subtypes: some patients have peripheral denervation (neuropathic POTS), some have symptoms that are due to sustained or parosyxmal overactivity of the sympathetic nervous system-increased amount of catecholamines increase the blood pressure upon standing (hyperadrenergic POTS) and some individuals have POTS dominated by features of deconditioning. Management of POTS includes avoidance of precipitating factors, volume expansion, physical countermaneuvers, exercise training, pharmacotherapy, pressure garments (abdominal binders, compression stockings)and behavioral-cognitive therapy. Therapies for POTS are targeted at relieving low blood volume or regulating circulatory problems that could be causing the disorder. Simple interventions such as adding extra salt to the diet and attention to adequate fluid intake (1.5-2 L) are also often effective. Increasing salt is an effective way to raise blood pressure in many patients with orthostatic hypotension by helping the body retain water and thereby expanding blood volume. Physical countermaneuvers, such as leg crossing, bending forward and placing a foot on a chair, making a fist, or active contraction of abdominal or buttock muscles may produce small increases in mean arterial pressure to maintain an adequate cerebral blood flow and prevent fainting. As in all causes of physical deconditioning, reduced stroke volume is a key component in the pathogenesis of POTS. All exercise programs for POTS patients should begin with low-intensity exercises for a short duration and progress slowly, gradually increasing the regimen over the next 6 to 8 weeks. Pharmacotherapy includes the mineralocorticoid fludrocortisone which promotes intravascular volume expansion through increasing sodium retention, the $\alpha 1$-adrenergic agonist midodrine which elicits peripheral vasoconstriction and reduces venous pooling, β-blockers propranolol, bisprostol which control the excessive sinus tachycardia, and the cholinesterase inhibitor pyridostigmine which prolongs the phasic effects of acetylcholine on the autonomic ganglia, leading to peripheral sympathetic vasoconstrictor output (and potentiating vagal effects) on standing [35]. Through slowing down the tachycardia, β-blockers, leading with propranolol, make the heart more efficient by increasing the time spent in diastole, thus allowing more time for the left ventricle to fill with blood. They also inhibit the release of renin from the juxtaglomerular apparatus in the kidneys which decreases the amount of circulating aldosterone with decrease result of blood volume due to increased sodium excretion. However, they also decrease blood pressure by decreasing the heart rate and myocardial contractility. Raj et all. showed in their study that at low doses, propranolol reduces standing heart rate and improves orthostatic symptoms and in higher doses it can more effectively control tachycardia, but do not improve quality of life or orthostatic symptoms, moreover it can worsen it. [36] Arnold et al. conducted the study to determine the effect of low-dose propranolol on maximal exercise capacity in patients with postural tachycardia syndrome [37]. According to their results it was suggested that propranolol, when used at low doses, may provide a modest beneficial effect to improve heart rate control and exercise capacity in POTS. Although direct comparison of β-blockade and exercise has not been conducted, it has been suggested that exercise is more effective for treatment in POTS. Endurance exercise training reduces standing heart rate, increases blood volume, cardiac mass, and exercise capacity; and improves quality of life.

Propranolol Use in Epilepsy

For a long time it has been suspected that epilepsy and cardiac arrhythmia may have common molecular background. Seizures can affect function of the central autonomic control centers leading to alterations of cardiac rhythm. In general, cardiac arrhythmias appear in up to 42% of all epileptic patients. Numerous studies have demonstrated anticonvulsant effects of antiarrhythmic drugs. Among beta-blockers (class II), propranolol showed anticonvulsant features in models for generalized tonic-clonic and complex partial seizures, but not for myoclonic convulsions. Many of β-blockers have direct membrane-stabilizing effects related to Na^+ channel blockade, like some classical antiepileptic drugs such as phenytoin, carbamazepine, valproate as well as newer ones (felbamate, lamotrigine, oxcarbazepine, topiramate, zonisamide). Luchowska et al. conducted the study in which theyinvestigated the efficacy of valproate, diazepam, phenytoin and carbamazepine, administered together with β-blockators, against generalized tonic-clonic seizures in mice [38]. According to their result propranolol and metoprolol might enhance the anticonvulsant potential of valproate and diazepam, but they do notchange the antiepileptic potential of carbamazepine and phenytoin.

Atenolol, does not affect the anticonvulsive activity of any of these antiepileptics. Propranolol and metoprolol are highly lipophilic agents, easily penetrating to the brain, and on the other hand atenolol very poorly enters the brain, consistently, atenolol did not influence the activity of anticonvulsants. This might indicate that the observed effect of propranolol and metoprolol's administration is mediated at the central level.

Fischer in his study also presented results in which it was shown that propranolol and its two enantiomers have anticonvulsant effects for generalized tonic–clonic and complexpartial seizures [39]. Through the study it was suggested that the sodium channel blocking properties and not the ß-receptor antagonistic activity accounts for the anticonvulsant effects of propranolol.

Propranolol Use in Sympathetic Storming After Severe Traumatic Brain Injury

Propranolol is also used in sympathetic storming after severe traumatic brain injury which occurs usually within the first 24 hours after severe traumatic brain injury or up to weeks later. The outward expressions include hypertension, hyperthermia, pupillary dilatation, tachycardia, cardiac arrhythmias, profuse sweating, an increased release of glucose, and an increased basal metabolic rate.

It is estimated that this exaggerated stress response occurs in 15% to 33% of patients with severe traumatic brain injury who are comatose (score on Glasgow coma scale ≤ 8).Theories on the cause of the episodes range from loss of cortical control over autonomic function (Hortnag et al.), loss of physiological regulatory mechanisms (Klug et al.), disinhibitory control of sympathetic outflow (Bullard), disruption of the autonomic relay system (Boeve et al.) to dysregulation of the autonomic nervous system. If the episodes are associated with severe hypertension and tachycardia, propranolol can be used due to the fact that it suppresses sympathetic outflow, slowing neuronal activity. It also decreases serum levels of catecholamines, reduces cardiac workload and inhibits central fevers by acting directly within the central nervous system. Dosing starts at 10 mg twice a day and is adjusted upward with doses as high as 640 mg per day reported [40].

Conclusion

In conclusion, indications for propranolol use in neurology are essential tremor, prophylaxis of migraine, postural tachycardia syndrome, sympathetic storming after severe traumatic brain injury and enhancement of antiepileptic drug potential.

Abbreviations

AAN = American Academy of Neurology
AHS = American Headache Society
EFNS = European Federation of Neurological Societies

References

[1] Olesen J, Hougard K, Hertz M: Isoproterenol and Propranolol: Ability to Cross the Blood-Brain Barrier and Effects on Cerebral Circulation in Man; *Stroke*, Vol 9, No 4.

[2] Elble RJ, Tremor Research Group. Report from a U.S. conference on essential tremor. *Mov. Disord*. 2006;21(12):2052–61.

[3] Louis ED, Ferreira JJ. How common is the most common adult movement disorder? Update on the worldwide prevalence of essential tremor. *Mov. Disord* 2010; 25: 534–41.

[4] Rajput AH, Offord KP, Beard CM, Kurkland LT. Essential tremor in Rochester, Minnesota: a 45-year study. *J. Neurol. Neurosurg. Psychiatry* 1984; 47: 466–70.

[5] Gulcher JR, Jonsson P, Kong A, et al. Mapping of a familial essential tremor gene, FET1, to chromosome 3q13. *Nat. Genet*. 1997; 17: 84–87.

[6] Higgins JJ, Loveless JM, Jankovic J, Patel PI. Evidence that a gene for essential tremor maps to chromosome 2p in four families [erratum in Mov Disord 1999; 14: 200]. *Mov. Disord*. 1998; 13: 972–77.

[7] Louis ED, Zheng W, Jurewicz EC, et al. Elevation of blood - carboline alkaloids in essential tremor. *Neurology* 2002; 59: 1940–44.

[8] Louis ED, Jurewicz EC, Applegate L, et al. Association between essential tremor and blood lead concentration. *Environ Health Perspect* 2003; 111: 1707–11.

[9] Louis ED, Faust PL, Vonsattel JP, Honig LS, Rajput A, et al. (2007) Neuropathological changes in essential tremor: 33 cases compared with 21 controls. *Brain* 130: 3297–3307.

[10] Axelrad JE, Louis ED, Honig LS, Flores I, Ross GW, et al. (2008) Reduced Purkinje cell number in essential tremor: a postmortem study. *Arch. Neurol*. 65: 101–107.

[11] Shill HA, Adler CH, Sabbagh MN, Connor DJ, Caviness JN, et al. (2008) Pathologic findings in prospectively ascertained essential tremor subjects. *Neurology* 70: 1452–1455.

[12] Chung SJ, Kwon H, Lee D-K, Hong JY, Sunwoo M-K, et al. (2013) Neuroanatomical Heterogeneity of Essential Tremor According to Propranolol Response. *PLoS ONE* 8(12): e84054.

[13] Koller WC, Vetere-Overfield B (1989) Acute and chronic effects of propranolol and primidone in essential tremor. *Neurology* 39: 1587–1588.

[14] Cleeves L, Findley LJ (1984) Beta-adrenoreceptor mechanisms in essential tremor: a comparative single dose study of the effect of a non-selective and a beta-2 selective adrenoreceptor antagonist. *J. Neurol. Neurosurg. Psychiatry* 47: 976–982.

[15] Calzetti S, Findley LJ, Gresty MA, Perucca E, Richens A (1981) Metoprolol and propranolol in essential tremor: a double-blind, controlled study. *J. Neurol. Neurosurg. Psychiatry* 44: 814–819.

[16] Baker MR, Baker SN (2012) Beta-adrenergic modulation of tremor and corticomuscular coherence in humans. PLoS One 7: e49088.

[17] Hoshi E, Tremblay L, Feger J, Carras PL, Strick PL (2005) The cerebellum communicates with the basal ganglia. *Nat. Neurosci*. 8: 1491–1493.

[18] Critchley M. Observations on essential tremor (heredofamilial tremor). Brain 1949; 72: 113–39.

[19] Rajput AH, Rozdilsky B, Ang L, Rajput A. Significance of Parkinsonian manifestations in essential tremor. *Can. J. Neurol. Sci* 1993; 20: 114–17.

[20] Zesiewicz TA, Elble R, Louis ED, et al. Practice parameter: therapies for essential tremor: report of the Quality Standards Subcommittee of the American Academy of Neurology. *Neurology* 2005; 64: 2008–20.

[21] Ferreira J, Sampaio C. Essential tremor. Clin Evid 2005;13: 1608–21.

[22] Abila B, Wilson JF, Marshall RW, et al. The tremorolytic action of betaadrenoceptor blockers in essential, physiological and isoprenaline-induced tremor is mediated by beta-adrenoceptors located in a deep peripheral compartment. *Br. J. Clin. Pharmacol.* 1985;20(4):369–76.

[23] Koller WC, Vetere-Overfield B. Acute and chronic effects of propranolol and primidone in essential tremor. *Neurology* 1989; 39: 1587–88.

[24] Larsen TA, Teräväinen H. Larsen TA, Teräväinen H. Beta 1 versus nonselective blockade in therapy of essential tremor. *Adv. Neurol.* 1983;37:247–51.

[25] Use of botulinum neurotoxin for the treatment of movement disorders. AAN summary of evidence-based guidelines for clinicians. 2008.

[26] Loder E, Burch R, Rizzoli P: The 2012 AHS/AAN Guidelines for Prevention of Episodic Migraine: A Summary and Comparison With Other Recent Clinical Practice Guidelines /Headache 2012;52:930-945.

[27] Hazard E, Munakata J, Bigal ME, Rupnow MF, Lipton RB. The burden of migraine in the United States: current and emerging perspectives on disease management and economic analysis. *Value Health*. 2009;12(1):55-64.

[28] Headache Classification Subcommittee of the International Headache Society (2004). "The International Classification of Headache Disorders: 2nd edition". *Cephalalgia* 24 (Suppl 1): 9–160.

[29] Silberstein SD, Freitag FG. Preventative treatment of migraine. *Neurology.* 2003;60(7):S38-44.

[30] Kowacs PA, Piovesan EJ, Tepper SJ. Rejection and acceptance of possible side effects of migraine prophylactic drugs. *Headache.* 2009;49(7):1022-27.

[31] Silberstein SD, Dodick DW, Lindblad AS, Holroyd K, Harrington M, Mathew NT, Hirtz D: Randomized, placebo-controlled trial of propranolol added to topiramate in chronic migraine /Neurology 78 March 27, 2012.

[32] Freeman R., Wieling W., Axelrod F.B. Consensus statement on the definition of orthostatic hypotension, neurally mediated syncope and the postural tachycardia syndrome. *Clin. Auton. Res.* 2011;21(2):69–72.

[33] Hermosillo, A. G.; Jordan, JL; Vallejo, M; Kostine, A; Márquez, MF; Cárdenas, M (2006). "Cerebrovascular blood flow during the near syncopal phase of head-up tilt test: A comparative study in different types of neurally mediated syncope". Europace 8 (3): 199–203.

[34] Parsaik A.T., Allison T.G., Singer W. Deconditioning in patients with orthostatic intolerance, *Neurology.* 2012.

[35] Benarroch EE: Postural Tachycardia Syndrome: A Heterogeneous and Multifactorial Disorder, *Mayo Clin. Proc. Dec* 2012; 87(12): 1214–1225.

[36] Raj SR, Black BK, Biaggioni I, et al. Propranolol decreases tachycardia and improves symptoms in the postural tachycardia syndrome: less is more. *Circulation* 2009;120:725–734.

[37] Arnold AC, Okamoto LE, Diedrich A, Paranjape SY, Raj SR, Biaggioni I, Gamboa A: Low-dose propranolol and exercise capacity in postural tachycardia syndrome/ *Neurology* 80 May 21, 2013

[38] Luchowska E, Luchowski P, Wielosz M, Kleinrok Z, Czuczwar SJ, Urbanska EM: Propranolol and metoprolol enhance the anticonvulsant action of valproate and

diazepam against maximal electroshock/ Pharmacology, *Biochemistry and Behavior* 71 (2002).

[39] Fischer W: Anticonvulsant profile and mechanism of action of propranolol and its two enantiomers/ *Seizure* 2002; 11: 285–302.

[40] Kishner S, Augustin J, Strum S. Post head injury autonomic complications. Available at: www.emedicine.com/pmr/topic108.htm.

In: Propranolol
Editor: Mislav Puljević

ISBN: 978-1-63482-974-8

Chapter 9

Propranolol: A Protective Mechanism for Bone Marrow Dysfunction Following Injury

Alicia M. Mohr, MD, FACS, FCCM[1,*]
and Ines G. Alamo, MD, MPH[2]
[1]University of Florida/Department of Surgery-
Associate Professor of Surgery, Gainesville, FL, US
[2]University of Florida/Department of Surgery-
Lab Researcher, Gainesville, FL, US

Abstract

Severely injured trauma patients develop persistent anemia that lasts for weeks following their initial injury. In these critically ill patients, there is a prolonged hypercatecholamine state. Both epinephrine and norepinephrine (NE) are elevated and this sustained elevation of catecholamines is associated with bone marrow (BM) dysfunction. Specifically, high concentrations of NE have been shown to directly suppress BM hematopoietic progenitor cells (HPCs) growth. In addition, NE induces HPC mobilization into the peripheral blood.

Both suppression of BM HPC growth and loss of HPCs into the peripheral blood are associated with BM dysfunction that manifests as a persistent injury-associated anemia.

Propranolol, a nonselective beta-blocker (BB), has been shown to prevent HPC growth suppression in the BM and as well as decrease mobilization of HPC into the peripheral blood. In our rodent injury and shock models, optimal therapeutic dose and timing of propranolol was also determined. In particular, early administration of at least 5 mg/kg of propranolol immediately following resuscitation is required to maintain BM cellularity, protect BM HPC growth and prevent HPC mobilization.

* Corresponding author: Alicia M. Mohr MD, FACS FCCM. Associate Professor of Surgery, University of Florida, Department of Surgery, 1600 SW Archer Road, Box 100108, Gainesville, FL 32610. Tel: (352) 273-5670, fax: (352) 273-5683, e-mail: alicia.mohr@surgery.ufl.edu.

Based on available rodent data, the benefit of early propranolol administration among severely injured trauma patients was also investigated. The goal of the study was to evaluate the potential therapeutic hematologic benefit that propranolol may provide in resolving this anemic state.

A prospective, randomized control study was performed, in which patients, following a traumatic injury were evaluated for eligibility. Among the propranolol-treated group, there was a significant decrease in HPC mobilization into the peripheral blood. Specifically, two markers of mobilization of HPCs in the peripheral blood, colony-forming unit erythroid cells (CFU-E) and blast-forming unit erythroid cells (BFU-E), were markedly decreased by 50% on day 1 and propranolol treatment maintained a 80-90% decrease on day 14 as compared with the untreated control groups. Furthermore, there was a clinically significant increase in hemoglobin (Hb) between those treated with propranolol (9.9± 0.4 g/dL) as compared to untreated controls (9.1 ± 0.6 g/dL).

Persistent injury-associated anemia is associated with BM dysfunction, which is accompanied by a hypercatecholamine state. Early propranolol administration following injury protects the BM from depletion of HPCs and can potentially prevent the use of late blood transfusions and improve this injury-related anemia. Future larger clinical studies are necessary to further elucidate the hematologic benefits of this therapy.

Introduction

Critical acute injuries in trauma patients, such as severe tissue injury and hemorrhagic shock (HS), are associated with an overwhelming stimulation of the sympathetic drive. Specifically, the sympathetic nervous system releases a vast amount of catecholamines, including epinephrine and norepinephrine (NE). Acutely, such an abundant response from the sympathetic nervous system is warranted in this setting. Physiological reactions such as increased blood pressure and heart rate (HR) are necessary to battle severe trauma and injury. However, this response persists longer in severely injured trauma patients who demonstrate a prolonged catecholamine elevation.

This prolonged stimulation is associated with bone marrow (BM) dysfunction, cardiovascular dysfunction, metabolic breakdown, and immune dysfunction [1]. Trauma-induced hypercatecholaminemia plays a critical role in BM dysfunction and it is associated with a persistent injury-associated anemia [2]. Previous work has shown that high concentrations of NE mediate a prolonged mobilization of HPCs into peripheral blood from the BM [3, 4]. HPCs play a key role in red blood cell production and erythropoiesis. NE controls the early release of HPC into the peripheral blood. Both the prolonged mobilization of HPCs in combination with the blunted HPC growth in BM after severe injury contributes to BM dysfunction [3, 5]. This trauma-induced hypercatecholaminemia is associated with persistent anemia in the clinical setting, which can last for several months after the initial injury and it is not related to acute blood loss [6]. Persistent injury-associated anemia often leads to multiple blood transfusions, which have been shown to be a strong independent predictor of infections, multiple organ failure, and mortality [7, 8]. Despite implementations to restrict transfusions in the intensive care unit (ICU), severely injured patients continue to receive blood transfusions that prolong their hospital stay and contributes to morbidity.

Regulation of the excessive catecholamine release in severely injured trauma patients has been examined previously. Particularly, beta blockade (BB) has shown improved outcomes in patients with acute brain injury, acute respiratory distress syndrome (ARDS), and burn injuries [9-12]. Patients with acute brain injuries have catecholamine overstimulation, which has been associated with increased risk of neurogenic cardiac dysfunction such as stress cardiomyopathy [12].

However, exposure to BB for at least two days in these patients was associated with decreased mortality when compared to patients who did not receive BB. Similarly after severe burns, patients remain in a catabolic state, which leads to loss of lean body mass and muscle wasting [9]. Long term BB administration decreased lean-mass catabolism among these patients [9]. The effects of propranolol, a nonselective beta-blocker, on clinically relevant models such of trauma, including lung injury and HS, has also demonstrated some hematologic benefits [3]. Propranolol given in an injury and shock model has been shown to prevent HPC mobilization to the periphery, allow HPC retention in the BM for improved BM cellularity and HPC growth, and lead to higher hemoglobin (Hb) levels [3].

In addition, propranolol exerts its BM protective effect in a dose and time dependent fashion. Early propranolol administration after severe injury is most therapeutic.

In this chapter, the role of hypercatecholamine state in BM dysfunction will be defined. In severely injured trauma rodent models, there is a clinically relevant environment of trauma-induced hypercatecholaminemia. In delineating the strong influence NE has on BM function, we will also demonstrate the significant role propranolol plays as a regulator of catecholamine response and restoration of BM function. This will be explained through research done in both injury and shock rodent models as well as in severely injured trauma patients. This chapter will also demonstrate a clinical application of propranolol therapy among severely injured trauma patients. The use of propranolol therapy was evaluated for its ability to limit the administration of blood transfusions, and treatment of BM dysfunction. The reversal of BM dysfunction can lead to beneficial hematologic outcomes.

Trauma-Induced Hypercatecholaminemia and Bone Marrow Dysfunction

In rodent models of injury as well as in trauma patients, severe injury has been proven to lead to significant BM dysfunction [13-15]. Severe tissue injury and hemorrhagic shock (HS) results in significant shifts in BM hematopoiesis and is associated with persistent injury-associated anemia [13]. Normal hematopoiesis in the BM is a complex and highly regulated activity that allows for proliferation and differentiation necessary for maturation of blood and immune cells [14]. In order for this highly regulated activity to function appropriately, HPCs must cooperate with multiple types of cells including progenitor, immune, and stromal cells, also found in the BM.

Under normal conditions, there is a steady state of homing and egress between the BM and the peripheral circulation. Homing is a process where cells migrate to the organ of their origin; in this case, it is the BM for HPCs. Egress is a process where cells move out of the organ of their origin and into the circulation.

Both homing and egress occur continuously at a low steady state under homeostatic conditions. Environments that disrupt this normal BM activity include severe trauma such as tissue injury and HS, inflammatory states, chemotherapy, and radiation [14]. In previous work with severe tissue injury and HS models, prolonged BM dysfunction was observed in part due to the mobilization of HPCs from the BM to the periphery to the site of injury. At the site of injury, these cells were trapped, inhibiting cells to return to the BM; hence, contributing to the prolongation of BM dysfunction [14].

This is similar to what is seen in an ischemic myocardium. In an ischemic myocardium, stem cells leave the BM and migrate to the area of ischemia for myocardial repair, causing a significant imbalance of stem cells BM to periphery ratio, thus, disrupting the homeostatic environment [16]. NE is a key regulator of mobilization and homing of HPCs with the BM [15]. Beta-2 adrenergic stimulation by NE resulted in increased numbers of circulating HPCs [15] Thus, high concentrations of NE inhibit BM HPC growth and also significantly prolonged HPC mobilization [15, 16].

Within the BM, there are multiple mediators that are involved in the proliferation and maturation of erythroid progenitor cells, including erythropoietin, catecholamines, and cytokines [3]. However, overstimulation of the key mediators can overwhelm and disrupt the homeostatic normal erythropoietic process in the BM. In the BM, both mature and immature cells express alpha and beta-adrenergic receptors [3]. In normal hematopoiesis, beta-adrenergic receptors have a stimulatory effect on the growth of normal progenitor cells. The influence of trauma-induced hypercatecholaminemia on BM hematopoiesis is key in the development of persistent injury-associated anemia. Although the surge of stress caused by trauma stimulates the releases of both catecholamines, NE and epinephrine (EPI), it is mainly NE that causes the disruption of normal hematopoiesis in the BM [15-17]. NE has dose dependent effects on BM HPC growth both in vivo and in vitro [17]. Under physiologic conditions, NE stimulates BM HPC growth *in vitro* [18]. However, as the concentration of NE increases, there is significant suppression of BM HPC growth [18]. Similarly, the inhibitory effect of NE on BM HPC growth *in vivo* was also evaluated. In this *in vivo* model, NE infused via an osmotic pump led to significant BM HPC growth suppression (Figure 1) [18].

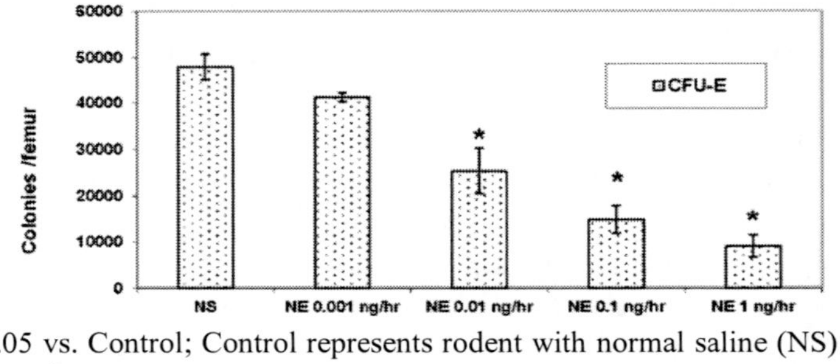

(n=6/group). *P<0.05 vs. Control; Control represents rodent with normal saline (NS) in osmotic pump; X axis: concentration.

Figure 1. NE has a concentration dependent effect on CFU-E growth in vivo.

The role of NE in BM dysfunction was further investigated in a more clinically relevant animal model. Combining severe tissue injury and HS in a rodent model a more severe traumatic injury was created [3]. Rodent models were assigned to severe tissue injury alone or severe tissue injury with HS and were euthanized at 24 hours and 7 days post injury. To recreate severe tissue injury, lung contusion was performed by using a blast wave of a percussive nail gun, which was applied to a 12-mm small metal plate on the right axilla of the rat [3]. For the HS model, HS was reached by withdrawing blood to a mean atrial pressure of

30 to 40 mmHg for 45 minutes. At the end of the 45 minutes, rats were resuscitated with reinfusion of the shed blood.

In the tissue injury only model, 50% BM HPC growth suppression was noted post injury on day 1 but only 15% reduction by day 7. However, the combination of severe tissue injury and HS led to a more severe and persistent BM HPC growth suppression (50 to 70%) by day 7 (Figure 2A) [3]. In addition, the addition of propranolol (BB) completely restored BM CFU-E growth on day 7 (Figure 2B). Based on these research outcomes, two vital observations were noted: a) NE is a crucial key mediator of BM dysfunction and b) its' impact is related to the degree of injury. In addition to the direct effects on BM, NE also causes HPC mobilization. Previous work has shown that the surge of catecholamines causes an increase of metalloproteinases and a decrease of stromal cell-derived factor 1 (SDF-1), a key gatekeeper in maintaining HPCs in BM for adequate growth and maturation [19].

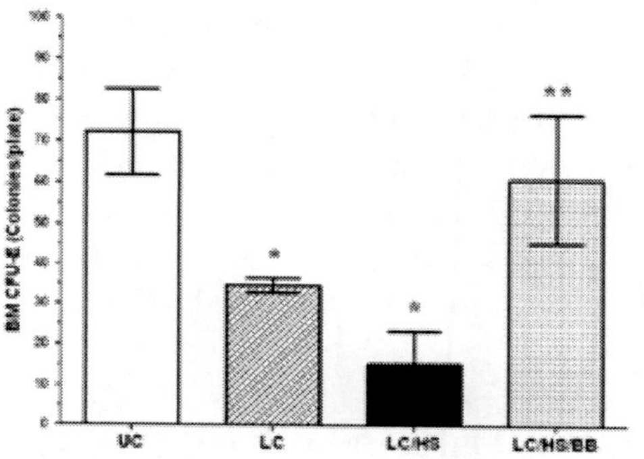

a

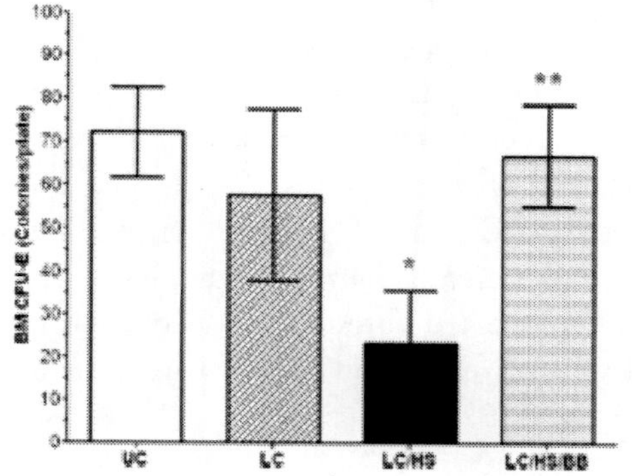

b

(n=4-6/group) UC=Naïve, LC/HS/BB=LCHS followed by BB after resuscitation'. *P<0.05 vs UC; **P< 0.05 vs. LCHS.

Figure 2. BM CFU-E colony growth at day 1 (A) and day 7 (B) after severe tissue injury and HS.

This shift causes HPC mobilization from the BM [19]. In our models, severe tissue injury alone and tissue injury combined with HS, both caused significant HPC mobilization from the BM to the periphery [3]. The mechanism that drives HPC mobilization is carried out by granulocyte colony stimulating factor (G-CSF), a potent stimulator [15]. NE mediates the release of G-CSF. Thus prolonged elevation of NE is associated with persistent elevation G-CSF and ongoing loss of HPCs to the peripheral blood [5]. Severe tissue injury and HS cause an initial stress response that stimulates the sympathetic nervous system to react with a release of catecholamines as part of the essential fight or flight response.

This response is appropriate and necessary in an acute setting. The problem lies when the release of catecholamines is sustained which occurs during inflammation and environments of chronic stress after severe tissue injury and HS [20]. The continued presence of high levels of NE leads to a prolonged release of HPCs from the BM and directly suppresses BM HPC growth. The combination of direct suppression and excessive release of HPCs leads to significant BM dysfunction. Hence, the severity and duration of BM dysfunction following severe traumatic injury is dependent on the persistence of adrenergic stress [3].

BM dysfunction with prolonged HPC mobilization from the BM and prolonged BMHPC growth suppression is associated with injury-associated persistent anemia [2, 6, 7]. In the combined severe tissue injury and HS model, on Day 7, hemoglobin (Hb) levels were significantly lower than the naïve controls and those with tissue injury alone (Figure 3) [3].

Among severely injured trauma patients, injury-associated anemia develops as early as day 3 and continued for several weeks post initial injury, in absence of any blood loss [21]. Previous work on severely injured trauma patients demonstrated that the supporting BM stroma failed to grow in over 90% of the patients and these patients had a corresponding mean Hb concentration of 8.6 ± 1.0 g/dL [6]. Persistent injury-associated anemia is a clinical manifestation of BM dysfunction that is impacted by the duration of trauma-induced hypercatecholaminemia.

The Protective Role of Propranolol

With the discovery of the substantial role NE played on BM dysfunction following severe trauma, the focus shifted on how to alleviate its effects. Beta-adrenergic receptor blockade (BB) with non-selective BBs have shown to be beneficial in patients with burn, trauma, non-cardiac operations, and traumatic brain injuries [9-12]. The use of non-selective BB with propranolol resulted in increased wound healing among burn patients and improved epithelialization as compared to untreated burn patients.

In addition, the propranolol-treated burn patients had a shorter hospital stay compared to the untreated group (24±8 vs 31±8 days) and required significantly less skin grafting (13.8% vs 18.7% total body surface area) [22].

	UC	LC	LC/HS	LC/HS/BB
WBC (10^3/µl)	7.3±2	6±2	5.2±1	7.8±2
RBC (10^6/ µl)	7.2±0.3	6.9±0.5	5.3±0.9*	6.7±0.5**
Hb (g/dL)	14.4±0.9	13.6±0.5	10.2±1.7*	13.4±0.8**
MCV (fl)	59±2	57±2	56±1	58±2

(N = 4-6/group) UC=unmanipulated control; LC=lung contusion; LC/HS=lung contusion followed by hemorrhagic shock; LC/HS/BB=LC/HS followed by beta blockade after resuscitation WBC=white blood cell; RBC=red blood cell; Hb=hemoglobin; MCV=mean corpuscular volume. *P<0.05 vs. UC; **P<0.05 vs. LC/HS.

Figure 3. Peripheral blood hematologic parameters seven days after injury.

With regard to trauma, in a lung injury rodent model, the use of propranolol prior to lung injury prevented BM HPC growth suppression. To determine which beta adrenergic receptors were involved with this BM protection, additional studies with selective beta-1 (B1), beta-2 (B2), and beta-3 (B3) blockers given prior to lung injury demonstrated that BM protection was mediated through the B2 and B3 blockers [23].

Propranolol therapy was then tested in the HS rodent model. Results mirrored what was found with the lung injury rodent model. Propranolol protected BM HPC growth whether it was administered prior or immediately after HS [24]. Propranolol administration among the HS rodent models was not associated with increased mortality rate or significant changes in blood pressure. The effectiveness of propranolol dosing was associated with a decrease in HR. The decrease of HR averaged approximately 20 %. It is also important to note that dose studies of propranolol use demonstrated that the safe range of IP (intraperitoneal) propranolol injections in rats ranged between 0.5mg/kg to 20mg/kg. However, 10mg/kg was chosen because it was believed to exhibit a physiologic effect without risking higher mortality [24].

Utilizing a more clinically significant model of combined lung contusion with HS, propranolol was administered, IP at 10mg/kg, immediately after resuscitation and was given daily for seven days. In this combined injury and shock model, there is significant 50-70% BM growth suppression at seven days. With the addition of daily propranolol post injury and shock, HPC growth was significantly increased.

In addition, there was restoration of Hb levels to near normal with the use of propranolol in this model. There are several models including rodent footshock stress model, murine hypoxia, and acute blood loss which demonstrate significant increases in RBCs or Hb levels with the use of propranolol [3, 25, 26].

While HPC mobilization is necessary for tissue healing, the persistent egress of HPCs seen with a hyperadrenergic state is detrimental. Along with preserving BM function, propranolol use prevented the prolonged mobilization of HPCs to the site of injury. When examining histologically the injured lung tissue, lung injury scores (LIS) can be quantified. Quantified LIS accounts for inflammatory cells, interstitial edema, pulmonary edema, and alveolar integrity and ranges between zero and eleven [27]. Use of propranolol following injury and shock did decrease both HPC mobilization in peripheral blood as well as HPC growth in injured tissue. In addition, the use of propranolol did not worsen wound healing (Figure 4) [3]. This finding is supported by studies that demonstrate that the use of BB in wound healing actually improves epithelialization and wound healing [22, 28].

In our clinically relevant model of lung injury and HS, propranolol provided BM protection. Propranolol prevented the suppression of BM HPC growth and reduced HPC mobilization to the peripheral blood without worsening lung healing. However, to truly evaluate the potential clinical application of propranolol, an effective dose and time of the therapeutic window of propranolol was investigated [29].

For these studies, combined lung injury and HS rodent models were used. To evaluate the effects of different dosages, rodent models of lung injury and HS received propranolol at the following doses: 1, 2.5, 5, or 10mg/kg dose via IP injection after resuscitation and daily for six days [29].

In respect to dose response effects on the bone marrow, we found that daily treatments of 5 and 10 mg/kg of propranolol significantly provided BM protection by preserving BM cellularity and also preventing prolonged BM HPC growth suppression (Figure 5A and 5B) [30].

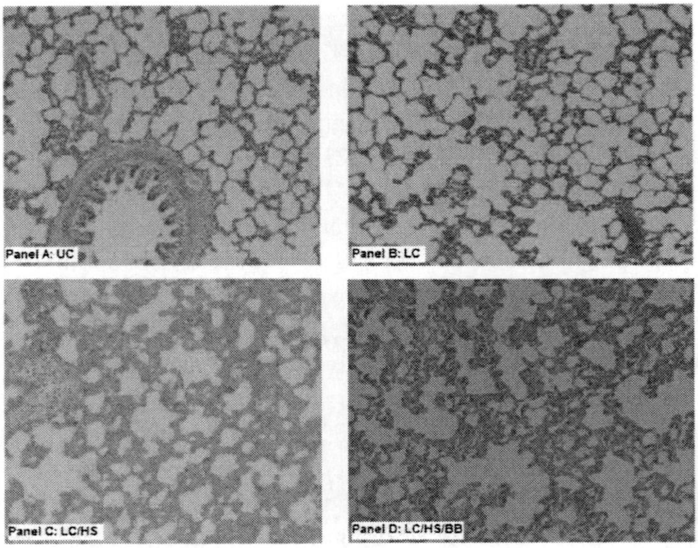

UC=Naïve, LC/HS/BB=LCHS followed by BB after resuscitation.

Figure 4. Histological differences of the contused lung tissue on Day 7 when compared with uninjured lung (A: UC). Almost healed contused lung (B: LC). Delayed healing at Day 7 illustrated with the addition of HS to LC (C). BB use did not worsen LIS (D).

Lower doses of propranolol did not sufficiently provide BM protection because of the severity of trauma-induced hypercatecholaminemia noted in these models; hence, a higher dose is more effective. It is also important to note that there is a significant 20% decrease in HR between the tissue injury and HS models that received propranolol versus non-treated groups [29].

Although propranolol's protective role is facilitated by B2 and B3 receptors, the effect of decreased HR provided by B1 in propranolol is a valuable marker in guidance for effective dosing of propranolol therapy in a clinical setting [29].

Previous work of propranolol used HR as a marker for optimal therapy in reducing hypermetabolism and for wound healing in burn patients [9, 22].

Both studies demonstrated that propranolol doses that effectively decreased HR by 20% was associated with therapeutic effects.

To determine the optimal therapeutic window, IP 10mg/kg of propranolol was given at various time points following resuscitation post HS [29].

Propranolol was either administered immediately, one hour, and three hours after resuscitation. These groups of animals were sacrificed three hours after propranolol was administered. The optimal therapeutic window for propranolol administration was one-hour post resuscitation following lung injury and HS model. Within this hour, BM function is preserved and HPC mobilization is inhibited (Figure 6).

Administration beyond one hour, propranolol lost its protective effect on the BM [29]. Similarly, following thermal injury in rats, vagal stimulation within thirty minutes after injury offered protection from lung injury [30].

Clinical Applications of Propranolol and Injury-Associated Persistent Anemia in Trauma Patients

Blood transfusion is part of the resuscitation protocol following acute traumatic injury. However, severely injured trauma patients who receive blood transfusions in the first 24 hours after injury have a high risk of developing persistent injury-associated anemia [8]. Subsequent blood transfusions are a strong independent predictor for mortality, incidence of multi-organ failure (MOF), infection, length of stay (LOS) in the ICU setting and overall hospital stay [8]. What remains concerning is that trauma patients tend to receive blood transfusions at a frequent rate; previous work has shown that overall blood transfusion rates were as high as 19.4% among trauma patients [8].

Blood transfusions also are associated with stimulation and prolongation of an inflammatory response due to the incubation of normal neutrophils with plasma from stored blood [31, 32]. This inflammatory response is further enhanced in acute severe trauma setting which prolongs the hypercatecholamine state which is associated with a persistent anemia.

Therefore, efficacious alternatives to blood transfusions are important in these patients. With the discovery of propranolol and its protective actions to preserve BM function and HPC growth, clinical applications were warranted. Propranolol use was then studied in a severely injured trauma patient population.

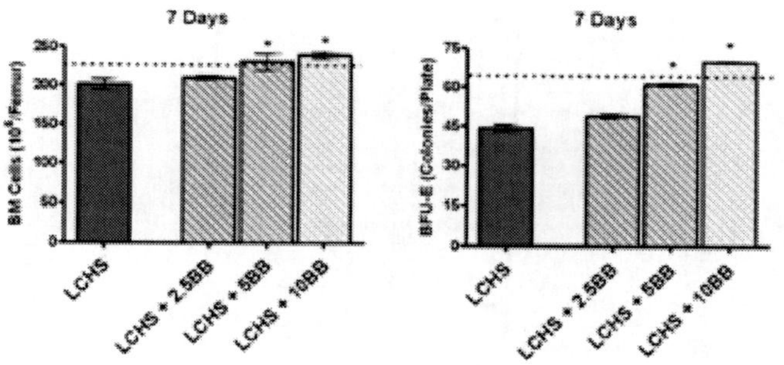

a b

Dotted line=Naïve control. *P<0.05 vs LCHS.

Figure 5. Continuous suppression of BM cellularity continued at Day 7 (5A) along with decreased BM HPC growth (5B) when compared to naïve levels. Again, a dose of BB at least 5 mg/kg, there is preservation of BM cellularity and HPC growth.

Therapeutic Window Bone Marrow and Peripheral Blood Parameters						
		BM HPC colony growth				
	BM Cellularity (cells x 10^6/femur)	CFU-GEMM (colonies/plate)	BFU-E (colonies/plate)	CFU-E (colonies/plate)	CD 71+/CD 117+ cells (% in PB)	Plasma GCSF (pg/mL)
UC	223 ± 12	37 ± 3	64 ± 3	72 ± 3	0.11 ± 0.07	5 ± 0.5
LCHS alone	126 ± 22	10 ± 1	23 ± 3	12 ± 3	13.88 ± 7.81	214 ± 178
LCHS+BB PR	289 ± 45*	34 ± 0*	67 ± 1*	65 ± 2*	0.04 ± 0.03*	35 ± 20*
LCHS+BB 1hr PR	227 ± 7*	31 ± 2*	56 ± 1*	60 ± 1*	0.38 ± 0.23*	176 ± 97
LCHS+BB 3hr PR	157 ± 13	13 ± 3	30 ± 4	33 ± 4	8.62 ± 1.10	215 ± 102

(n=4-10 per group). *P<0.05 vs. LCHS.

Figure 6. BB given immediately after resuscitation and at one hour maintains BM cellularity and BM HPC growth, prevents HPC mobilization, and elevation of G-CSF.

In a prospective, randomized, controlled study of forty-five trauma patients treated at a Level One Trauma Center the effects of propranolol on BM function was performed [2]. All patients who participated in the study underwent a traumatic injury and were enrolled within twenty-four hours of admission (Figure 7) [2].

Among these forty-five patients, twenty were randomly assigned as the untreated group while the rest, twenty-five, were assigned to the propranolol treated group. The dosing was based on a titration to cause a 10% to 20% decrease in the average initial HR [2]. If this decrease was not reached within thirty minutes, the patient received an additional 0.5 mg intravenously and HR was rechecked.

This dosage increase of 0.5 mg occurred every six hours until the targeted HR was achieved. It is important to note that if a patient's HR dropped to less than 60 beats per minute or mean arterial pressure was less than 50 mm Hg, the following dose was held and additional doses were lowered by one algorithm level [2]. Blood was collected on all patients participating in the study on admission and a time course (Day 1, 5, 10, 14, and 30 post initial injuries) pending upon discharge. Unless a patient was discharged, intervention was concluded after thirty days. Highlighted patient characteristics included mean age of patients was 33 years old, mean injury severity score (ISS) was twenty-nine, and 36% presented in shock (Figure 8) [2]. The rest of the patient demographic breakdown is noted in Table 3.

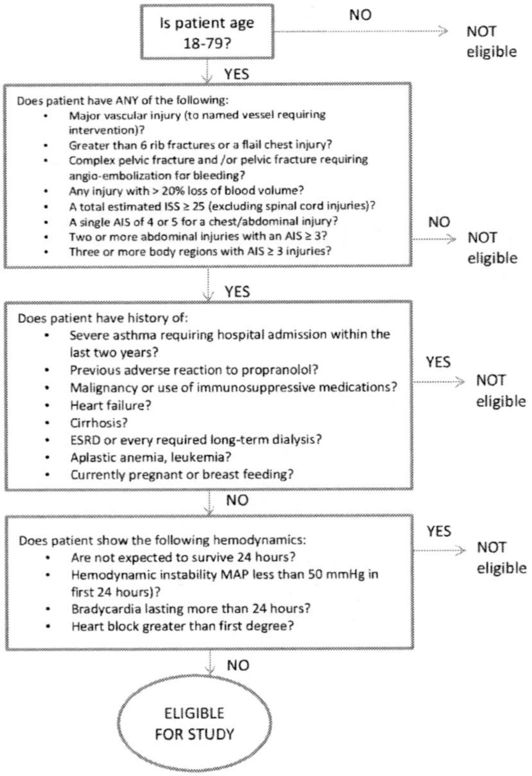

ISS=injury severity score; AIS=abbreviated injury score; ESRD=end stage renal disease; MAP=mean arterial pressure.

Figure 7. Diagram of inclusion and exclusion criteria.

Characteristic	Control	Propranolol	P value
N	20	25	
Male/Female	20/0	19/6	<0.05*
Age, y	30 ± 7	35 ± 7	0.18
Ethnicity:			
Black (%)	14 (70)	17 (68)	0.89
Caucasian (%)	6 (30)	8 (47)	
Mechanism of injury:			
Blunt (%)	4 (20)	15 (60)	<0.05*
Penetrating (%)	17 (80)	10 (40)	
ISS	31±3	27±3	0.31
Admission base deficit	-7.4±1.5	-7.4±1.4	0.99
Lactate (mg/dL)	6±1	5±1	0.26
Initial heart rate, bpm	111±6	104±4	0.47
Initial SBP, mmHg	108±7	113±6	0.38
Admission GCS	14±1	13±1	0.33

ISS=injury severity score; SBP=systolic blood pressure; GCS=Glasgow coma scale; *P <0.05.

Figure 8. Demographic data by group.

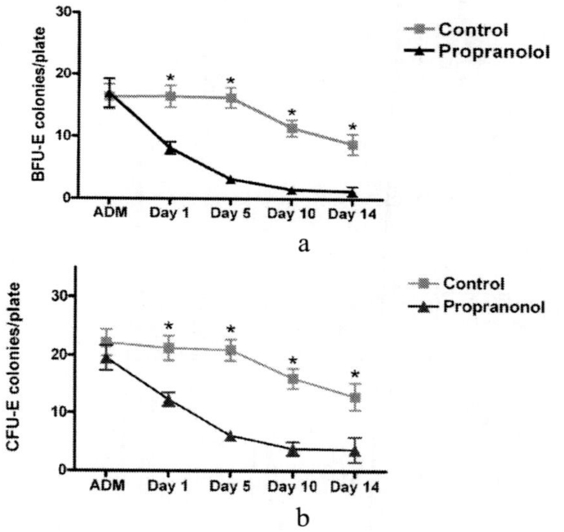

*P <0.05.

Figure 9. The effect of propranolol therapy on HPC mobilization. (A) BFU-E growth in peripheral blood in each group on admission (ADM) and at each time point (Days 1, 5, 10, and 14). (B) CFU-E growth in peripheral blood in each group on ADM and at each time point (Days 1, 5, 10, and 14).

Dosing was effective in two-thirds of the treated patients. Compared to the untreated group, HR and MAP were lower among the propranolol treated group [2]. On the day of admission, significant HPC mobilization into the peripheral blood was noted in both groups of patients. In untreated group, HPC mobilization remained significantly elevated from Day 1 to Day 14 (Figures 9A and 9B). This further supports previous data that HPC mobilize after severe acute injury [33]. In contrast, on Day 1, the propranolol treatment group demonstrated a significant decrease in colony forming unit-erythroid (CFU-E), in the peripheral blood (Figure 9A and 9B). The beneficial effects of propranolol were seen from Day 1 until Day 14. These data clearly shows that early propranolol treatment prevents HPC mobilization.

Similarly, trauma-induced hypercatecholaminemia mediates the release of G-CSF, which led to the prolonged mobilization of HPCs into the periphery. In both groups, plasma G-CSF was markedly elevated on admission. G-CSF remained elevated in the untreated group until the day of discharge (Figure 10). Comparably, the propranolol treated group demonstrated a 51% decrease in G-CSF on Day 1. On Day 10, G-CSF decreased 90% with propranolol treatment as compared to the untreated group [2].

Throughout their stay in the hospital, all patients developed a persistent injury-associated anemia. However, our work demonstrated that with the use of propranolol, there is a potential medical therapy for anemia following trauma.

On the day of discharge, there is a clinical increase in Hb levels between the untreated and propranolol treated groups (9.9 ± 0.4 g/dL versus 9.1 ± 0.6 g/dL) [2].

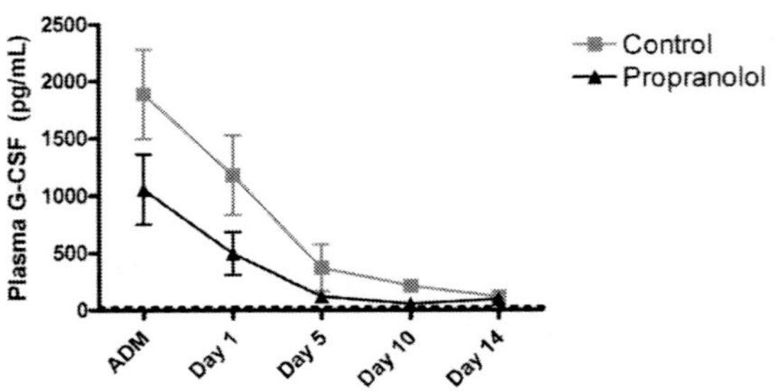

G-CSF=granulocyte-colony stimulating factor.

Figure 10. Effect of propranolol therapy on G-CSF levels on ADM and at each time point (Days 1, 5, 10, and 14).

	Control		Propranolol	
	Hemoglobin g/dL (95%CI)	Reticulocyte count % RBCs (95%CI)	Hemoglobin g/dL (95%CI)	Reticulocyte count % RBCs (95%CI)
Admission	12.2±0.4 (11.3-13)	1.2±0.2(0.9-1.5)	12.2±0.5 (11.2-13.0)	1.2±0.1 (0.9-1.4)
Day 1	9.8±0.3 (9.1-10.5)	1.7±0.1 (1.4-1.9)	10.2±0.5 (9.2-11.2)	1.5±0.2 (1.2-1.8)
Day 5	8.6±0.3 (8.1-9.3)	2.7±0.3 (2.1-3.2)	9.2±0.6 (8.4-9.9)	2.7±0.2 (2.2-3.1)
Day 10	8.8±0.4 (8-9.6)	3.1±0.4 (2.5-4.1)	9±0.4 (8.1-9.8)	3.5±0.3 (2.9-4.1)
Day 14	9.1±0.4 (8.4-9.9)	3.3±0.4 (2.6-4)	8.9±0.5 (7.9-9.7)	4.0±0.6 (2.8-5.3)
Discharge	9.1±0.6 (8.4-10.3)	3.3±0.3 (2.9-3.9)	9.9±0.4 (8.6-10.4)	4.6±0.4 (3.7-5.0)

RBCs=red blood cells.

Figure 11. Effect of propranolol therapy on hematologic parameters on admission and at each timepoint (day 1, 5, 10, and 14) until discharge.

There was no difference in number of blood transfusions to account for this difference.

Furthermore, although both groups demonstrated an increase over time in reticulocyte count, an indicator of production of RBCs, the rate of increase was higher in the propranolol treated group (Figure 11). This study is the first to evaluate the potential use of propranolol therapy to improve BM dysfunction and improve persistent injury-associated anemia following trauma. This study demonstrates that the early use of propranolol therapy is safe and prevents HPC mobilization and provides a potential faster resolution of anemia following severe trauma.

When propranolol is administered early and in titrated doses aimed to reduce HR by 10 to 20% from initial baseline values, this drug was both safe and effective. Based on this work, further clinical investigations are necessary in providing further insight on the benefits of propranolol can provide in severely injured trauma patients in the setting of injury-associated anemia.

Conclusion

Severely injured trauma patients undergo acute, normal physiological responses in order to compensate for initial injury. If the stress is continued, the sympathetic nervous system continues to be stimulated. The potency of this noradrenergic overstimulation causes prolonged HPC mobilization and persistence BM HPC growth suppression which results in BM dysfunction. This presents clinically as persistent injury-associated anemia. This persistent anemia often leads to the overuse of blood transfusions, which makes patients vulnerable to increased risk of infection, organ failure, and death.

Throughout this chapter, we have outlined the roles of three specific key mediators in the development of persistent injury-associated anemia. Severe trauma, trauma-induced hypercatecholaminemia, and overstimulation of B2 and B3 BM receptors mediated by NE all play an instrumental role in BM suppression. Like mentioned before, BM suppression appears as a result of premature HPC mobilization from the BM to the periphery to site of injury which leads to BM HPC growth suppression.

Out of the three mediators mentioned, the initial injury is the factor that can be controlled the least. In the ICU, tissue injury and HS trigger an overwhelming inflammatory response. Severe physiological inflammatory responses from such injuries ignite key mediators such as catecholamines, specifically NE. NE mediates the release of G-CSF, which activates the mobilization of HPC from the BM to the periphery. This egression of premature HPCs into the periphery prevents BM HPC growth and eventually leads to BM dysfunction. This BM dysfunction is best manifested as injury-associated anemia among trauma patients.

The continuous cycle of events described above were delineated throughout this chapter along with a potential medical therapy: propranolol. Propranolol is a nonselective beta-blocker that inhibits B2 and B3 receptors, prevents HPC mobilization from the BM and prevents BM growth suppression. There are limitations to our clinical findings, but these findings are relevant and the first of its kind. Further clinical relevant trials are necessary to evaluate the hematologic protection propranolol can provide for trauma patients with injury-associated anemia.

References

[1] Godbout, J. P., Glaser, R. Stress-induced immune dysregulation: implications for wound healing, infectious disease and cancer. *Journal of neuroimmune pharmacology: the official journal of the Society on NeuroImmune Pharmacology*. 2006;1:421-7.

[2] Bible, L. E., Pasupuleti, L. V., Alzate, W. D., Gore, A. V., Song, K. J., Sifri, Z. C., et al. Early propranolol administration to severely injured patients can improve bone marrow

dysfunction. *The journal of trauma and acute care surgery*. 2014;77:54-60; discussion 59-60.

[3] Mohr, A. M., ElHassan, I. O., Hannoush, E. J., Sifri, Z. C., Offin, M. D., Alzate, W. D., et al. Does beta blockade postinjury prevent bone marrow suppression? *The Journal of trauma*. 2011;70:1043-9; discussion 9-50.

[4] Fonseca, R. B., Mohr, A. M., Wang, L., Clinton, E., Sifri, Z. C., Rameshwar, P., et al. Adrenergic modulation of erythropoiesis following severe injury is mediated through bone marrow stroma. *Surgical infections*. 2004;5:385-93.

[5] Cook, K. M., Sifri, Z. C., Baranski, G. M., Mohr, A. M., Livingston, D. H. The role of plasma granulocyte colony stimulating factor and bone marrow dysfunction after severe trauma. *Journal of the American College of Surgeons*. 2013;216:57-64.

[6] Livingston, D. H., Anjaria, D., Wu, J., Hauser, C. J., Chang, V., Deitch, E. A., et al. Bone marrow failure following severe injury in humans. *Annals of surgery*. 2003; 238: 748-53.

[7] Bateman, A. P., McArdle, F., Walsh, T. S. Time course of anemia during six months follow up following intensive care discharge and factors associated with impaired recovery of erythropoiesis. *Critical care medicine*. 2009;37:1906-12.

[8] Malone, D. L., Dunne, J., Tracy, J. K., Putnam, A. T., Scalea, T. M., Napolitano, L. M. Blood transfusion, independent of shock severity, is associated with worse outcome in trauma. *The Journal of trauma*. 2003;54:898-905; discussion-7.

[9] Herndon, D. N., Hart, D. W., Wolf, S. E., Chinkes, D. L., Wolfe, R. R. Reversal of catabolism by beta-blockade after severe burns. *The New England journal of medicine*. 2001;345:1223-9.

[10] Arbabi, S., Ahrns, K. S., Wahl, W. L., Hemmila, M. R., Wang, S. C., Brandt, M. M., et al. Beta-blocker use is associated with improved outcomes in adult burn patients. *The Journal of trauma*. 2004;56:265-9; discussion 9-71.

[11] Auerbach, A. D., Goldman, L. beta-Blockers and reduction of cardiac events in noncardiac surgery: clinical applications. *JAMA*. 2002;287: 1445-7.

[12] van der Jagt, M., Miranda, D. R. Beta-blockers in intensive care medicine: potential benefit in acute brain injury and acute respiratory distress syndrome. *Recent patents on cardiovascular drug discovery*. 2012;7:141-51.

[13] Livingston, D. H., Gentile, P. S., Malangoni, M. A. Bone marrow failure after hemorrhagic shock. *Circulatory shock*. 1990;30:255-63.

[14] Badami, C. D., Livingston, D. H., Sifri, Z. C., Caputo, F. J., Bonilla, L., Mohr, A. M., et al. Hematopoietic progenitor cells mobilize to the site of injury after trauma and hemorrhagic shock in rats. *The Journal of trauma*. 2007;63:596-600; discussion -2.

[15] Katayama, Y., Battista, M., Kao, W. M., Hidalgo, A., Peired, A. J., Thomas, S. A., et al. Signals from the sympathetic nervous system regulate hematopoietic stem cell egress from bone marrow. *Cell*. 2006;124:407-21.

[16] Orlic, D., Kajstura, J., Chimenti, S., Bodine, D. M., Leri, A., Anversa, P. Bone marrow stem cells regenerate infarcted myocardium. *Pediatric transplantation*. 2003;7 Suppl. 3: 86-8.

[17] Penn, A., Mohr, A. M., Shah, S. G., Sifri, Z. C., Kaiser, V. L., Rameshwar, P., et al. Dose-response relationship between norepinephrine and erythropoiesis: evidence for a critical threshold. *J. Surg. Res*. 2010;163:e85-90.

[18] Fonseca, R. B., Mohr, A. M., Wang, L., Sifri, Z. C., Rameshwar, P., Livingston, D. H. The impact of a hypercatecholamine state on erythropoiesis following severe injury and the role of IL-6. *The Journal of trauma*. 2005;59:884-9; discussion 9-90.

[19] Spiegel, A., Shivtiel, S., Kalinkovich, A., Ludin, A., Netzer, N., Goichberg, P., et al. Catecholaminergic neurotransmitters regulate migration and repopulation of immature human CD34+ cells through Wnt signaling. *Nature immunology*. 2007;8:1123-31.

[20] Molina, P. E. Neurobiology of the stress response: contribution of the sympathetic nervous system to the neuroimmune axis in traumatic injury. *Shock*. 2005;24:3-10.

[21] Shander, A. Anemia, Erythropoeitin, and the Trauma. *Patient Trauma Care*. 2008;18: 29-34.

[22] Mohammadi, A. A., Bakhshaeekia, A., Alibeigi, P., Hasheminasab, M. J., Tolide-ei, H. R., Tavakkolian, A. R., et al. Efficacy of propranolol in wound healing for hospitalized burn patients. *Journal of burn care and research: official publication of the American Burn Association*. 2009;30:1013-7.

[23] Beiermeister, K. A., Keck, B. M., Sifri, Z. C., ElHassan, I. O., Hannoush, E. J., Alzate, W. D., et al. Hematopoietic progenitor cell mobilization is mediated through beta-2 and beta-3 receptors after injury. *The Journal of trauma*. 2010;69:338-43.

[24] Elhassan, I. O., Hannoush, E. J., Sifri, Z. C., Jones, E., Alzate, W. D., Rameshwar, P., et al. Beta-blockade prevents hematopoietic progenitor cell suppression after hemorrhagic shock. *Surgical infections*. 2011;12: 273-8.

[25] Lucian, H. Effects of beta-adrenergic receptor blockade on stress-induced changes in hematological parameters of rats. *Turkish Society of Hematology* 2006;23:90-3.

[26] Zyuz'kov, G. N., Abramova, E. V., Dygai, A. M., Gol'dberg, E. D. Role of adrenergic mechanisms of erythropoiesis regulation during severe hypoxia. *Bulletin of experimental biology and medicine*. 2005;140:13-7.

[27] Claridge, J. A., Enelow, R. I., Young, J. S. Hemorrhage and resuscitation induce delayed inflammation and pulmonary dysfunction in mice. *J. Surg. Res*. 2000;92:206-13.

[28] Silvamani, R. Stress-Mediated Increases in Systemic and Local Epinephrine Impair Skin Wound Healing: Potential New Indication for Beta Blockers. *Plos Med*. 2009;6.

[29] Baranski, G. M., Offin, M. D., Sifri, Z. C., Elhassan, I. O., Hannoush, E. J., Alzate, W. D., et al. beta-blockade protection of bone marrow following trauma: the role of G-CSF. *J. Surg. Res*. 2011;170:325-31.

[30] Song, X. M., Li, J. G., Wang, Y. L., Liang, H., Huang, Y., Yuan, X., et al. Effect of vagus nerve stimulation on thermal injury in rats. *Burns: journal of the International Society for Burn Injuries*. 2010;36:75-81.

[31] Fransen, E., Maessen, J., Dentener, M., Senden, N., Buurman, W. Impact of blood transfusions on inflammatory mediator release in patients undergoing cardiac surgery. *Chest*. 1999;116:1233-9.

[32] Zallen, G., Offner, P. J., Moore, E. E., Blackwell, J., Ciesla, D. J., Gabriel, J., et al. Age of transfused blood is an independent risk factor for postinjury multiple organ failure. *American journal of surgery*. 1999;178:570-2.

[33] Claridge, J. A., Sawyer, R. G., Schulman, A. M., McLemore, E. C., Young, J. S. Blood transfusions correlate with infections in trauma patients in a dose-dependent manner. *The American surgeon*. 2002;68: 566-72.

In: Propranolol
Editor: Mislav Puljević

ISBN: 978-1-63482-974-8

Chapter 10

Propranolol As Chiral Agent

R. Čižmáriková*, J. Valentová and A. Némethy
Department of Chemical Theory of Drugs, Faculty of Pharmacy,
Comenius University in Bratislava, Bratislava, Slovak Republic

Abstract

This review deals with various chiral aspects of propranolol. Propranolol is an aryloxyaminopropanol-type β-adrenolytic drug, and is used as the standard that other β-blockers are generally compared with. In terms of β-adrenolytic activity, the (*S*)-(−)-enantiomer of propranolol is 100 times more effective than the (*R*)-(+)-isomer. In this chapter the pharmacodynamic, pharmacokinetic and toxicological effects of individual (*R*)-(+)- and (*S*)-(−)-enantiomers of propranolol are described, together with various methods for the chiral separation (HPLC, TLC, CE, TLC) of both enantiomers at both the analytical and preparative scale. Single (*R*)-(+)- and (*S*)-(−)-enantiomers with different levels of enantiomeric purity can be obtained using several methods of stereoselective synthesis.

Introduction

Propranolol (1-(isopropylamino)-3-(1-naphthyloxy)propan-2-ol.HCl) is the most well-known nonselective adrenergic antagonist that blocks the action of epinephrine and norepinephrine at both the β_1 and β_2 – adrenergic receptors. Propranolol has little intrinsic sympathomimetic activity (ISA), but has a strong membrane stabilizing effect (only at a high blood concentration, e.g. overdosage). This β-adrenergic blocker is widely used for various cardiovascular indications such as angina pectoris, hypertension [1] and post myocardial infarction treatment [2], as well as for mostly off-label extracardiovascular indications [3, 4] such as glaucoma [5], anxiety [6], migraine [7], and infantile hemangioma [8].

* Corresponding author: Email: cizmarikova@fpharm.uniba.sk.

British scientist James Black was awarded the Nobel Prize in Medicine for the discovery of propranolol [8].

Synthesis of (*R S*)-(±)-Propranolol

Propranolol **(Figure 1)** was derived from the early β-adrenergic antagonists of arylaminoethanol type, dichloroisoprenaline (dichloroisoproterenol) **(Figure 2)** and pronethalol **(Figure 3)**. The key structural modification, which was carried through to essentially all subsequent β-blockers, was the insertion of an oxymethylene bridge into the arylaminoethanol structure of pronethalol, thus greatly increasing the potency of the compound. This also apparently eliminated the carcinogenicity found with pronethalol in animal models. [10]

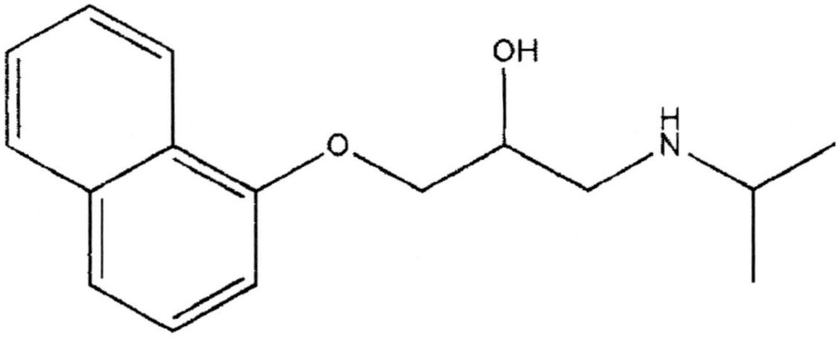

Figure 1. Propranolol.

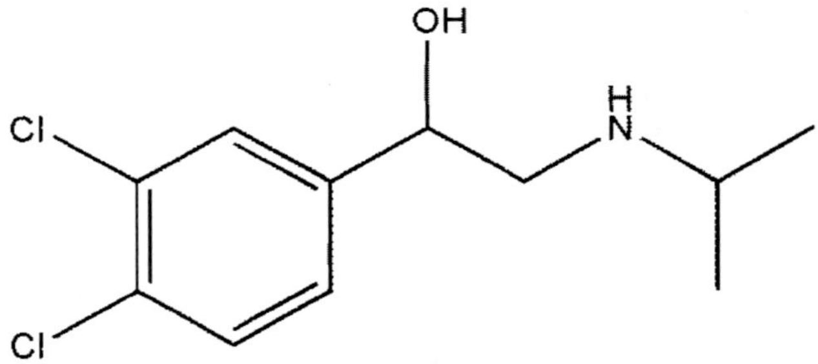

Figure 2. Dichloroisoprenaline.

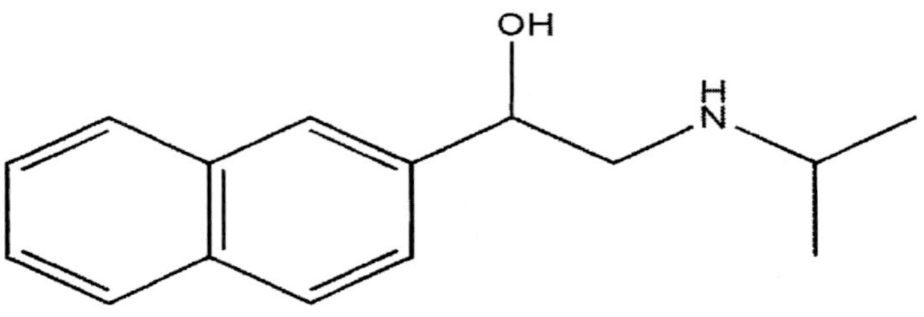

Figure 3. Pronethalol.

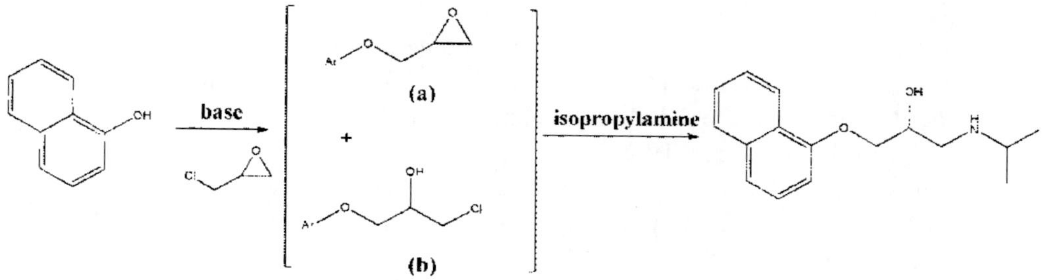

Figure 4. Synthesis of (±)-propranolol.

Propranolol is based on an aryloxyaminopropanol scaffold (as are its derivatives); it is synthesized in two steps from naphthalen-1-ol. Two products 2-[(1-naphthyloxy)methyl] oxirane **(Figure 4, a)** and different amount of 1-chloro-3-(1-naphthyloxy)propan-2-ol **(Figure 4, b)** were obtained by the reaction of naphthalen-1-ol with (±)-chloromethyloxirane. The reaction was carried out in an aqueous solution of a base (NaOH, KOH, K_2CO_3 etc.) or in organic solvent containing pyridine or piperidine with excess of chloromethyloxirane. Excellent yield of 2-[(1-naphthyloxy)methyl]oxirane was obtained by microwave activation using solid-liquid-free phase transfer catalyst [11].

Both intermediates react with isopropylamine and give a racemic base of propranolol **(Figure 4)** [12, 13]. Several methods have been published for the purpose of synthesizing racemic propranolol [14 - 16].

In the therapeutic practice, propranolol is used as a racemic salt with hydrochloric acid. This salt is white crystalline powder; odorless and has a bitter taste. It melts at about 164°C. It is soluble in water and in alcohol; slightly soluble in chloroform and practically insoluble in diethylether. Its molecular weight is 295.80 [12]. The structural differences between (*R S*)-propranolol hydrochloride and its (*S*)-enantiomer were further investigated by powder X-ray diffraction patterns, infrared spectra and solid-state NMR spectra. The solubility and metastable zone width of (*R S*)-propranolol hydrochloride in a mixed solvent of methanol and acetone were determined by cooling crystallization over the temperature range 3.5 - 42.5 degrees C [17].

The ternary solubility diagram of (*R*)-, (*S*)-propranolol hydrochloride was constructed using the same mixed solvent. The diagram will be useful as a guide for choosing crystallization operation conditions to produce pure enantiomers [18].

Enantiomers of Propranolol

Propranolol possess a stereogenic centre and can form different (*R*)-(+)- and (*S*)-(−)-enantiomers that are pairs of molecules for which the three-dimensional arrangement of atoms represents nonsuperimposable mirror images.

Enantiomers were distinguished by their ability to rotate the plane of polarized light. Isomers that rotate the plane of polarized light to the right, or in a clockwise direction, were designated as dextrorotatory and indicated by a (+)- sign before the chemical name [(+)-propranolol or (−)-propranolol]. The opposite designation, levorotatory or (−)-, was assigned to molecules that rotate the plane of polarized light to the left, or in a counterclockwise direction. The letters *d-* and *l-* were formerly used to indicate (+)- and (−)-, respectively. A racemate (racemic mixture) is 1:1 mixture of enantiomers and is indicated by placement of (±)- before the compound name. This nomenclature is based on a physical property of the molecule and does not describe the absolute configuration or three-dimensional arrangement of atoms around the chiral center [19-21].

Two enantiomers of propranolol can have different absolute configurations as designated by the Cahn-Ingold-Prelog (CIP) system, but the same relative orientation of the functional groups relevant for biologic activity [22, 23].

An example of this is demonstrated when the absolute configuration of the nonselective β-adrenergic antagonist propranolol is compared to norepinephrine **(Figure 5, 6)**. Because of the presence of the ether oxygen atom, the priority sequence of the functional groups about the chiral center results in the assignment of the (*S*)-absolute configuration for the more active enantiomer of propranolol. Close inspection of (*R*)-norepinephrine, (*R*)-pronethalol and (*S*)-propranolol, however, shows that the hydroxyl group, basic amine, and aromatic rings of both compounds occupy the same regions in three-dimensional space [20, 21].

Molecular modeling procedures are used for imaging of stereoselective interaction between aryloxyaminopropanol and receptors. This method allows viewing of 3D-structures of proteins and their binding sites using data from X-ray crystallography.

Several authors deal with searching for optimal ligand conformation and position of β-adrenergic blockers in cavities of β-receptors. In these papers flexible molecular docking analysis of interaction of β-adrenergic blockers in β-adrenergic receptor subtypes was used [24, 25]. Propranolol was studied at the serotonin receptors, also known as 5-hydroxytryptamine receptors or 5-HT receptors [26].

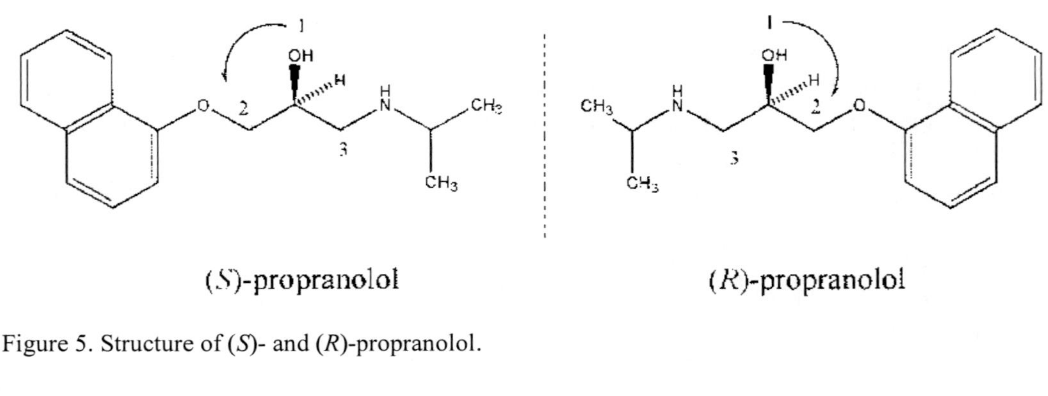

Figure 5. Structure of (*S*)- and (*R*)-propranolol.

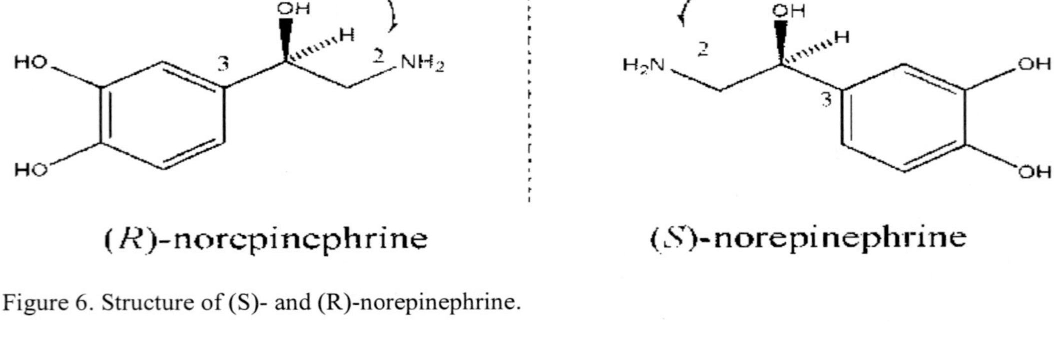

Figure 6. Structure of (S)- and (R)-norepinephrine.

Stereoselective Pharmacodynamics of Propranolol

When the enantiomers of propranolol are introduced into chiral environment such as the human body, they display different pharmacological and toxicological properties. The human body as a biological system is at a molecular level an intensely chiral environment being composed of macromolecules such as proteins, glycolipids and polynucleotides, consisting of the chiral building blocks of L-amino acids and D-carbohydrates.

As many of the processes of drug disposition and pharmacokinetics involve an interaction between the enantiomers of a drug molecule and a chiral biological macromolecule, it is hardly surprising that stereoselectivity is observed during this action [27].

The Easson-Stedman hypothesis states that the more potent enantiomer must be involved in a minimum of three intermolecular interactions with the surface of the biologic target and that the less potent enantiomer only interacts with two sites.

The three points of interaction of (*R*)-(−)-epinephrine (also for (*S*)-(−)-propranolol) with the receptor site are the aromatic ring, β-hydroxyl group, and the protonated secondary ammonium group. All three functional groups interact with their complementary sites on the receptor surface, resulting in receptor stimulation by epinephrine and receptor blockade by propranolol respectively.

The β-hydroxyl group of the opposite enantiomers is located in the wrong place in space and, therefore, cannot interact properly with the receptor.

This can lead to significant differences in their pharmacokinetic and pharmacodynamic behavior, resulting in adverse side effects or toxicity. For example, the individual isomers in a racemic mixture can exhibit significant differences in absorption (especially active transport), serum protein binding, and metabolism. As it relates to drug metabolism, it is certainly possible that only one of the isomers can be converted into a toxic substance or can influence the metabolism of another drug. Since stereochemistry can have a profound effect on both the pharmacokinetic and pharmacodynamic properties of a drug, it is important to review the foundational concepts [23, 28].

The major bioactive enantiomer, the eutomer, is (*S*)-(−)-propranolol, whose antiadrenergic effect is many times stronger than that of its less active distomer, the (*R*)-(+)-enantiomer, which manifests various adverse effects.

In the paper Stoschitzky et al. [29] the effects on forearm blood flow of brachial artery infusions of the (*R*)- and (*S*)- enantiomers of propranolol and atenolol (2, 10, and 50 micrograms/min each) and their inhibitory effects on isoprenaline-induced vasodilatation by forearm venous occlusion plethysmography in 12 healthy subjects were investigated. Results indicated that the optically pure (*R*)- and (*S*)-enantiomers of propranolol and atenolol do not exert direct vasoconstrictive effects. Furthermore, these results confirmed that predominantly (*S*)-enantiomers have β-adrenoceptor blocking effects, but they also showed that neither the non-β-blocking (*R*)-enantiomer of propranolol nor the (*S*)-enantiomer of the β_1-selective agent atenolol is completely devoid of blocking effects on vascular β_2-adrenoceptors.

The optical isomers of propranolol have been also compared for their β-blocking, antiarrhythmic and local anaesthetic activities. Barrett and Cullum obtained following results:

In blocking the positive inotropic and chronotropic responses to isoprenaline, (*R*)-(+)-propranolol had less than one hundredth the potency of (*S*)-(−)-propranolol. At dose levels of (*R*)-(+)-propranolol which attenuated the responses to isoprenaline, there was a significant prolongation of the *PR* interval of the electrocardiogram.

The metabolic responses to isoprenaline in dogs (an increase in circulating glucose, lactate and free fatty acids) were all blocked by (*S*)-(−)-propranolol. (*R*)-(+)-propranolol had no effect on fatty acid mobilization but significantly reduced the increments in both lactate and glucose.

Both isomers of propranolol possessed similar depressant potency on isolated atrial muscle taken from guinea-pigs.

The isomers of propranolol exhibited similar local anaesthetic potencies on an isolated frog nerve preparation at a level approximately three times that of procaine. The racemic compound was significantly less potent than either isomer. Both isomers of propranolol were capable of preventing norepinephrine-induced cardiac arrhythmias in cats anaesthetized with halothane, but the mean dose of (*R*)-(+)-propranolol was 0.09 ± 0.02 mg/kg whereas that of (*R*)-(+)-propranolol was 4.2 ± 1.2 mg/kg. At the effective dose level of (*R*)-(+)-propranolol there was a significant prolongation of the *PR* interval of the electrocardiogram. Blockade of arrhythmias with both isomers was surmountable by increasing the dose of epinephrine.

Both isomers of propranolol were also capable of reversing ventricular tachycardia caused by ouabain in anaesthetized cats and dogs. The dose of (*S*)-(−)-propranolol was significantly lower than that of (*R*)-(+)-propranolol in both species but much higher than that required to produce evidence of β-blockade [30].

Stereoselective Pharmacokinetics of Propranolol

Differences in the pharmacokinetics of propranolol enantiomers were observed in the drug's distribution (stereospecific bound to plasma proteins) and elimination (stereospecificity of liver enzymes). Stereoselective binding to β-adrenoceptor induces differences in pharmacodynamics. Propranolol is a basic drug that binds to both albumin and α_1-acid glycoprotein in the plasma.

For propranolol the stereoselective binding in both whole plasma as well as individual serum proteins has been reported. Stereoselectivity in the binding of propranolol to human serum, however, resembles that seen with α_1-acid glycoprotein.

A study of the propranolol binding in the maternal and fetal serum further confirmed the importance of α_1-acid glycoprotein in the overall extent of binding and stereoselectivity of propranolol significantly lower concentration of α_1-acid glycoprotein in the fetus blood (14 mg %) compared with that in the maternal blood (66 mg %) resulted in much higher free fraction and change in the direction of stereoselectivity in binding in the fetal blood [31, 32].

The tissue distribution of the enantiomers of propranolol has been reported using laboratory animals. Takahashi et al. demonstrated that, compared with the (+)-enantiomer, the (−)-enantiomer of propranolol reaches higher concentration in heart, muscle, gastrointestinal tract, kidney, brain, and lung of rat. However, this apparent stereoselectivity could be explained by higher free fraction of (*S*)-(−)-propranolol in plasma. Similarly, the stereoselective binding of the propranolol enantiomers to plasma proteins is the main reason behind an apparent stereoselectivity in the red blood cell distribution of the drug [33].

In man, propranolol is metabolized by three main pathways of ring hydroxylation, side chain oxidation and glucuronidation or sulfation respectively. The ring hydroxylation process may occur at either position four or five both of them showing substrate stereoselectivity for (*R*)-(+)-propranolol [34].

Authors characterized cytochrome P450 isozymes responsible for propranolol metabolism, especially N-desisopropylation and 5-hydroxylation, in human liver microsomes. These results indicate that propranolol 5-hydroxylation, as well as 4-hydroxylation, is mainly catalyzed by CYP2D6 in human liver microsomes [35].

The hydroxypropranolol is further conjugated with glucuronic acid, favoring the (*S*)-(−)-enantiomer, or sulphate, favoring the (*R*)-(+)-propranolol, before excretion into urine [36, 37]. The (*R*)-(+)-enantiomer is preferentially metabolized; the opposite is true at high propranolol concentration [34].

Various factors related to the drug (interaction between the enantiomers themselves and between the enantiomers and other drugs) and the patient (age, gender, disease states) may affect the stereospecific pharmacology of propranolol. These stereospecific pharmacokinetic and pharmacodynamic aspects of propranolol are published in the review [32].

Study of Other Stereoselective Activity of Propranolol

The (*R*)-(+)-enantiomer competes with (*S*)-(−)-propranolol for plasma protein binding sites, resulting in lower plasma protein binding of the (*S*)-(−)-enantiomer when the racemate is administered. From toxicological experiments, it was concluded that racemic propranolol is more toxic than the individual enantiomers in the rat, when dosed *i. v.* at the same total mass [38].

Differences of the individual enantiomers of propranolol were studied at the respiratory and cardiovascular function. Toet et al. studied the contribution of the enantiomers of propranolol to racemic propranolol intoxication in anaesthetized spontaneously breathing rats and artificially ventilated rats and rabbits. In the spontaneously breathing rats, as in artificially ventilated rabbits, the survival time in the (*R*)-(+)-propranolol group was significantly longer than in the racemic and (*S*)-(−)-propranolol group. In artificially ventilated rats survival times were not significantly different between the racemic, (*S*)-(−)- and (*R*)-(+)-propranolol group [39].

Acute and chronic studies were conducted with Daphnia magna and Pimephales promelas to determine enantiospecific toxicity of propranolol to a model aquatic invertebrate and vertebrate, respectively. Also, enantiospecific effects of propranolol on D. magna heart rate were examined. Acute (48-h) responses of both organisms were similar for all enantiomer treatments. Chronic P. promelas responses to propranolol enantiomers followed the hypothesized relationship of (*S*)-propranolol being more toxic than (*R*)-propranolol, but chronic D. magna responses did not. No enantiospecific effects on daphnid heart rate were observed in acute exposures [40].

Both enantiomers of propranolol have a local anaesthetic effect, which is normally mediated by blockade of voltage-gated sodium channel. In this study the biophysical effects of propranolol on recombinant heart and brain sodium channels were determined. It was found that the ability of propranolol to block voltage-gated sodium channels is not stereospecific, nor a class effect of β-blockers. These findings firmly establish sodium channels as targets for propranolol and may help explain some beneficial effects of the drug [41].

Racemic propranolol and its (*R*)-enantiomer inhibit sperm motility in a dose dependent manner. Spermicidal action depends upon its local anaesthetic properties rather than its β-blocking activity. The (*R*)-enantiomer, unlike the racemate, is devoid of the unwanted effects of β-blockade and thus may be a useful drug [42].

The influence of racemic propranolol compared to half dosed (*S*)-propranolol on the level of thyroid hormone level was investigated. The ratio of triiodothyronine to thyroxine was decreased by (*R, S*)-propranolol but not by (*S*)-propranolol, suggesting that only the (*R*)-enantiomer inhibits the conversion of thyroxine to triiodothyronine [43].

Suedee et al. studied differential permeation of propranolol enantiomers across human skin *in vitro*. When the pure enantiomers were used, there was a marked difference between the penetration rates of (*R*)- and (*S*)-propranolol. The permeation of the (*S*)-enantiomer was retarded. When racemic propranolol was used, the difference was reduced [44].

Propranolol and its two enantiomers have anticonvulsant effects in models for generalized tonic–clonic and complex partial seizures which may be accounted for by the sodium channel blocking and not by the ß-adrenoceptor blocking activity [45].

Stereoselective Chromatographic Analysis

The investigation of stereo selectivity in action and disposition of chiral drugs together with preparation of pure enantiomer drugs calls for efficient stereoselective analytical methods. Enantiomeric separation techniques based on chromatography have long been the method of choice in this respect. The chromatographic separation of propranolol has been used on preparative scale that provides rapid access to individual enantiomers [46].

There is also great demand for a method of enantiomers separation on an analytical scale for controlling synthesis, checking the racemization process, controlling chiral impurity of pharmaceuticals [47] and for pharmacokinetic and pharmacological studies [48, 49, 32]. Recently, stereoselective analysis of propranolol has been used for detection in environmental samples [50].

Different technologies have been used for enantioseparation of enantiomers on an analytical scale, such as high-performance liquid chromatography (HPLC), gas chromatography (GC), thin-layer chromatography (TLC), capillary electrophoresis (CE), and capillary electrochromatography (CEC).

The chiral separation of propranolol was often described within enantioseparation of beta-blockers group, however it was used in many cases as a model compound for study of new chiral selectors or mechanism of chiral separation. In earlier applications stereoisomers analysis was performed using ultraviolet (UV) and fluorescence detection (FLD), currently the liquid chromatography and mass spectrometry (LC-MS, LC-MS/MS) application are extending.

The strategies of chiral separation may be classified as direct or indirect. In an indirect separation the enantiomeric analytes are reacted with homochiral derivatizing reagent (CDA) to form a mixture of diastereoisomers which can be separated by conventional achiral chromatography. The direct separation is based on the formation of diastereoisomeric complexes between the enantiomeric analyte and a chiral selector in the system. The chiral selector is a part of mobile phase (chiral mobile phase additive - CMPA) or is bound to the chromatographic sorbent and created chiral stationary phase – CSP [51].

Gas Chromatography (GC)

Two strategies can be considered for the resolution of enantiomeric compounds by gas chromatography (GC). One method involves the conversion of enantiomers into diastereomeric derivatives with a proper auxiliary enantiomerically pure derivatization reagent prior to GC analysis. Another method for the resolution of enantiomers by GC takes advantage of chiral stationary phases [52].

Enantioseparation of racemic propranolol by gas chromatography requires a chiral derivatizing agent (*N*-heptafluorobutyryl anhydrid, *N,O*-bis(trimethylsilyl)trifluoroacetamide, trifluoroacetic anhydride, *N*-trifluoroacetyl-(*S*)-(-)prolylchloride), which converts enantiomers into diastereoisomers. The diastereoisomers differing in their physicochemical properties can hence generally be separated by conventional chromatographic columns [53, 54]. In the gas capillary chromatography the chiral stationary columns are mostly based on modified cyclodextrin [55].

In the paper Dönnecke et al., propranolol was separated using chiral stationary phase with 3-allyl-2,3-di-*O*-methyl-6-*O*-*terc*-butyldimethylsilyl-beta-cyclodextrin [56]. Abe et al. prepared the chiral column coated with (*S*)-valine-d-menthylamide-linked polysiloxane and propranolol was separated by this column at column temperature of 180 °C [57].

Propranolol and other aminoalcohols in the form of oxazolidin-2-ones derivatives were separated on the 18-m pyrex glass capillary column with the chiral stationary phase XE-60-l-valine-(*R*)-α-phenylethylamide [58].

In the paper Thomson et al. the derivatizing chiral reagent (*R*)- or (*S*)– phenylethyl isocyanate was examined. The reagent reacts exclusively with amino group even with a 100-fold excess of reagent [59].

Gas chromatography was also used to determine enantiomers of propranolol in the plasma and tissues [60, 61]. Enantiomers of propranolol and other ß -blockers such as diastereoisomer derivatives with *N*-trifluoroacetyl-1-prolyl-chloride, *N*-heptafluorobutyryl-1-prolyl-chloride and *N,O*-bis-(trimethylsilyl)trifluoroacetamide were separated on packed and glass open-tubular columns [62].

High-Performance Liquid Chromatography (HPLC)

Indirect Mode

This mode has some advantages, such as wide applicability, inexpensive achiral column packing, and enhancement detection, due to possibility of introducing additional chromophores or fluorophores. On the other hand, this method requires high optical purity of derivatizing reagents, and sometimes is laborious and time consuming [63]. Two functional groups of propranolol: amino and alcohol are target which are of use in diastereoisomer formation. A variety of derivatizing agents, including isocyanates and isothiocyanates [64, 65], chloroformates [66, 67], acylchloride acid [68] and anhydrides [69] were used for enantiomeric separation of propranolol and other beta-blockers.

Resently synthesised isothiocyanate chiral derivatizing agents: (1*S*, 2*S*)-*N*-[(2-isothiocyanato)-cyclohexyl]-pivalinoyl amide (PDITC), 2,3,4,6-tetra-*O*-acetyl-β-D-glucopyranosyl isothiocyanate (GITC) [70] and (1*R*,2*R*)-1,3-diacetoxy-1-(4-nitrophenyl)-2-propyl isothiocyanate [71] have been described for stereoanalysis of propranolol. Toyoka et al. implemented the derivatization by(*R*)-(-)-4-(3-isothiocyanatopyrrolidin-7-yl)-7-(*N,N*-dimethylaminosulfonyl)-2,1,3-benzoxadiazole (DBD-PyNCS) following separation of created stereoisomers on a reversed –phase column for determination of propranolol enantiomers in rat plasma and saliva [72, 73].

One of new derivatizing reagents was prepared by substitution of the fluorine atoms in 1,5-difluoro-2,4-dinitrobenzene (DFDNB) with three optically pure amines [(*R*)-(-)-1-cyclohexylethylamine, (+)-dehydroabietylamine and (*S*)-(-)-alpha,4-dimethylbenzylamine], with amino acid amides and amino acids. The formed diastereomers with propranolol were separated by RP-HPLC [74].

Enantioseparation of five β-blockers, namely, (*RS*)-atenolol, (*RS*)-propranolol, (*RS*)-bisoprolol, (*RS*)-metoprolol and (*RS*)-carvedilol, was achieved as their diastereomers prepared with chiral derivatizing reagents (CDRs) synthesized on a cyanuric chloride platform (6-methoxy derivative with amino acids or their amides). Separation of diastereomers was carried out on a C(18) column and gradient eluting mixtures of methanol with aqueous trifluoroacetic acid with UV detection at 230 nm [75].

It may be mentioned that *O*-glucuronide diastereoisomers of propranolol are formed naturally during the metabolism. Yu et al. [76] developed the simple RP-HPLC method using reversed ODS column with mixture of the phosphate buffer (pH 3.5) and methanol for direct determination (*R*)- and (*S*)-propranolol glucuronide in rat hepatic microsomes to investigate the stereoselectivity of propranolol glucuronidation metabolism.

Direct Mode

Chromatographic separation of enantiomers on chiral stationary phase has appeared as the most effective and convenient way of determining the enantiomeric composition of chiral drugs. Different structural type of CSPs including the derivatized polysaccharides [77, 13], proteins [78, 79], β-cyclodextrin [80, 81], π-donor/acceptor phases [82, 83], macrocyclic antibiotic [84, 85], and molecular imprinted phases [86] were utilized for enantiomeric separation of propranolol.

Polysaccharide-based stationary phase are the most widely used CSPs due to their high separation efficiency, selectivity, sensitivity and reproducibility and can be used under normal, reversed and polar organic phase modes [87]. Commercially available and the most used in the enantioseparation of ß -blockers are these derivatives cellulose tris-(3,5-dimethylphenylcarbamate) – Chiracel OD, Lux Cellulose 1, and amylose tris-(3,5-dimethylphenylcarbamate) – Chiralpak AD. The following molecular interactions are supposed to play role in chiral discrimination of enantiomers: H-bonding interaction with carbamate on CSP, π-π interaction with phenyl group on CSP and aromatic group of the solute, dipole-dipole interaction, and steric interaction [87, 88].

The molecular modelling studies of interaction of propranolol with cellulose tris-(3,5-dimethylphenylcarbamate) chiral selector demonstrated that the hydroxy group of propranolol is crucial in determining of stereochemistry of the structure. The position of the hydroxy group of (*R*)-enantiomer causes better affinity toward cellulose tris-(3,5-dimethylphenylcarbamate), strong bonds and it could be the main cause for its higher retention time compared to the (*S*)-enantiomer, allowing separation between enantiomers [89]. In the study Valentová et al. [90], enantiomers of propranolol and of some novel aryloxyaminopropanol derivatives with β-adrenoceptor antagonist activity were separated on Chiralpak AD CSP with final composition of mobile phase: *n*-hexane:ethanol: methanol:dimethylamine (85:3.75:11.25:0.1 %). The enantiomeric elution order was determined to be (*R*)- before (*S*)-enantiomer following semipreparative isolation and induced CD spectrum of complexes formed in situ with molybdenum tetraacetate.

The cellulose-(3,5-dimethylphenylcarbamate) CSP was used for semipreparative isolation of enantiomers of propranolol hydrochloride. The enantiomers were obtained using mobile phase system containing petroleum ether and propan-2-ol with basic additives [91].

Zhang et al. [92] performed enantiomeric separation of propranolol by reversed phase elution mode using Chiralpak AD-RH column for the enantioselective skin permeation.

Recently new immobilized CSP have become commercially available based on tris-(3,5-dimethylphenylcarbamate) of amylose and cellulose - Chiralpak IA, Chiralpak IB, and tris-(3,5-dichlorophenycarbamate) of cellulose - Chiralpak IC. Enantioseparation of ß -blockers involving propranolol on immobilized CSP (Chiralpak IA) was compared to the enantioseparation on coated CSP (Chiralpak). The coated phase showed a higher resolution power than the immobilized phase. However, the immobilized phase withstands solvents like dichloromethane when used as an eluent or as a dissolving agent for analyte [93]. The enantioseparation of propranolol on Chiralpak IB using a mobile phase consisting of *n*-hexane-ethanol-triethylamine (95:5:0.4%) and fluorescence detection was applied to the pharmacokinetic study of both enantiomers in rats. The serum concentration-time curve (AUC) of (*S*)-propranolol in rat serum after intraperitoneal administration was significantly higher than AUC of (*R*)-propranolol [89].

Macrocyclic antibiotic phases have recently been very useful group of chiral selectors for the separation of ß -blocker enantiomers. The commonly used macrocyclic antibiotics for chiral separations include teicoplanin, ristocetin, vancomycin and theiranalogues. These are used in organic or reversed phase mode and mobile phase is mostly consisted of acetonitrile, alcohols, and amines [63]. The enantioseparation might be achieved by several mechanisms (dipol, steric, and π-π interaction). The possible interactions between analytes strictly depend on mobile phase selection, which determines that enantiomers fit into the aglycone cavity [94].

The latest application using teicoplanine-based CSP in normal phase is analysis of propranolol enantiomer in highly contaminated river water, after solid phase extraction with molecularly imprinted polymers [50].

The vancomycine-based CSP (Chirobiotic V) in reversed phase was utilized in LC-MS method for enantioselective determination of propranolol in biological matrices (urine, plasma) [95] and in enviromental matrices (nature and waste water) [96, 97]. Ribeiro et al. [98] used Chirobiotic V under reversed mode in LC-MS/MS with a triple quadrupole analyser for identification of propranolol enantiomer beside other chiral pharmaceutical (beta blockers, beta2 adrenergic agonist, and selective serotonin reuptake inhibitors) in the effluents of wastewater treatment plants (WWTP). Monitor of chiral pharmaceutical in WWTP effluents has potential to assess the enantioselective biodegradation in bioreactors.

Bagnall et al. [99] presented first chiral liquid chromatography quadrupole time-of-flight mass spectrometry (LC-QTOF-MS) for analysis of enatiomers of propranolol and other drugs in river water and sewage eluent using separation on Chirobiotic V and CBH (cellobiohydrolase) column.

Some studies published enantioseparations of propranolol on **protein chiral stationary phases** base on α_1-acid glycoprotein (Chiral-AGP column) [100, 101] and cellobiohydrolase (chiral-BSH column) [102, 103]. One of the advantages of protein-base CSP column is possibility using an aqueous mobile phase and the fact that analyte derivatization is unnecessary. Many molecular interactions (e.g. hydrogen bond, π-π, dipole, and ionic) are believed to be involved in the complexation analytes due to the complexity of protein selector [87]. Xuan and Hage [104] investigated the effects of pH, temperature, ionic strength, and organic modifiers on retention and separation of propranolol enantiomers on the AGP column. It was found that change in the organic modifier concentration gave the largest change in retention and separation and that both coulombic and hydrophobic interactions played important roles in determining the retention of (*R*)- and (*S*)- propranolol.

Suegee et al. [105] performed an enantioselective assay of propranolol, pindolol and oxprenolol on an AGP column and the method was use for studying the release of enantiomers from dosage form.

Enantioseparation of propranolol on high selective **chiral stationary phase based on molecularly imprinted polymers** was also described [106]. Haginaka et al. [107], prepared molecularly imprinted polymer for (*S*)-propranolol using methacrylic acid and ethylene glycol dimethacrylate as a host functional monomer and cross linker, respectively. The prepared polymeric material had specific recognition for (*S*)-propranolol. Hydrophobic interaction of the naphthyloxy and propan-2-yl (isopropyl) groups of propranolol and ionic interaction of the propan-2-ylamino (isopropylamino) group of propranolol with the (*S*)-propranolol imprinted polymer are supposed to play an important role in enantioselective recognition of propranolol.

One of used direct methods for enantioseparation of propranolol and other drugs using **chiral mobile phase additive** as a chiral selector was described by Guillarme et al. [108]. They used columns packed with sub-2μm particles in liquid chromatography with very high pressure condition (UHPLC) and cyclodextrine directly added to the mobile phase. However, this strategy suffered from drawback linked to column lifetime and low enantioseparation efficiency. Better resolution of enantiomers was obtained by indirect mode after derivatization of analytes with Marfey's reagent and 2,3,4-tri-O-acetyl-α-D-arabinosyl isothiocyanate.

Stereoanalysis by Capillary Electrophoresis

In addition to the chromatographic methods, electrophoretic techniques have been used for enantioseparation of propranolol in recent years. Capillary electrophoresis (CE) has been selected for high separation efficiency, short analysis time, high resolving power, and low consumption of reagents [109, 110]. The direct approach, involving formation of reversible diastereomeric complexes of the enantiomers with different chiral selectors added to the backgroud electrolyte (BGE) or bonded to the stationary phase, is the method of choice to separate enantiomers.

Cyclodextrines (CDs) and their derivatives as chiral selectors are frequently used for enantioseparation due to their good solubility in aqueous buffers and wide availability [111, 112]. Enantiomers of propranolol were successfully separated using native CDs [113] and their derivatives, namely hydroxypropyl-β-CDs [114, 115], methyl β-CDs [116], and sulfated cyclodextrin [117]. Matthijs, 2006 et al. investigated the highly sulfated CDs (α,β,γ-HSCDs) for the determination of chiral impurity in pharmaceuticals containing propranolol and atenolol. Different experimental conditions were optimized to determine the enantiomeric impurity when it was eluted either before or after main compounds. Best separation conditions were obtained using phosphate buffer containing 5 % m/v of HS-α-CD [118]. Caboxymethyl-β-CDs, a negative chargeable CD, were used for simultaneous chiral analysis of propranolol and its metabolite 4-hydroxypropranolol [119].

In a nonaqueous CE system (NACE) for enantioseparation of ß blockers involving propranolol single isomer sulfated derivatives of CDs [120], heptakis (2,3-di-*O*-methyl-6-sulfo)-β-cyclodextrin (HDMS-β-CD), and heptakis (2,3-di-*O*-acetyl-6-sulfo)-β-cyclodextrin (HDAS-β-CD) were used as chiral agents [121 - 123]. The use of non-aqueous solvents in the BGE enhances hydrophobic analyte solubility and the method selectivity.

Enantiomers of propranolol were resolved in NACE system using ion paring agents: (-)-2,3,4,6-di-*O*-isopropylidene-2-keto-L-gulonic acid [124] and 1*S*,4*R*-(+)-ketopinic acid [125].

Several β-blocker involving propranolol were chirally separated by the ligand-exchange CE by di-n-amyl L-tartrate-boric acid complex [126] and Cu(II) complexes of L-tartaric acid and L-threonine. However, the enantiocapability of this method was poorer compared to the enantioseparation with CDs [127].

Among other chiral selectors in CE, human serum albumin [128, 129] and macrocylic antibiotics, namely clarithromycin lactobionate [130], sulfonated polysacharide χ-carragenan, and its sulfobutylether derivative [131, 132], were investigated for enantioseparation of propranolol. The novel chiral selector clindamycin phosphate, a lincosamide antibiotic, and a novel ternary complex of Cu(II)-clindamycin were evaluated for enantioseparation of propranolol based on the ligand exchange mechanism. In comparison with macrocyclic antibiotics, the complex posses high solubility and low UV absorption and therefore high-resolution [133].

Recently, other capillary electromigration techniques (MECK, MEEK, CEC, and MCE – microchip electrophoresis), novel chiral additives, and alternative detection (MS) for enantiomeric separation of propranolol have been introduced [134].

In MECK-micellar electrokinetic capillary chromatography, the chiral surfactants are added to an aqueous buffer and micelles are formed. The analyte is separated by its partitioning between the micelles, known as the chiral pseudostationary phase, and the buffer solution, known as the mobile phase. The main advantage of MECK is high resolution power for charged and uncharged compounds [112].

A number of novel polymeric surfactants for enatioseparation of propranolol by MECK were described such as polysodium *N*-undecenoxy carbonyl-L-leucinate (poly-L-SUCL) and *N*-undecenoxy carbonyl-L-isoleucinate (poly-L-SUCIL) [135]. In the study Rizvi et al. [136] propranolol with other six ß -blockers were separated in a single run by using different polymeric surfactants. Polysodium *N*-undecenoxy carbonyl amino acidate (poly-L-SUCAA) and polysodium *N*-undecenoxy-carbonyl amino acid sulphates (poly-L-SUCAASS). It was found that (poly-L-SUCAA) showed better resolution than the corresponding surfactants with sulfates group. Enantioseparation of propranolol using poly-L-SUCL coupled with MS detection singnificantly increased sensitivity of separation [137].

In chiral MEEK - Microemulsion micellar electrokinetic capillary chromatography, a chiral selector is usually component of the microemulsion, such as surfactants, cosurfactants and oils with chiral structure [138]. The chiral microemulsion for separation of propranolol enantiomer in MEEK method was prepared using eight different L-tartrates and D-tartrates with different alcohol moieties as chiral oils [139]. Other studies [140] used neutral microemulsion containing the surfactant Tween 20 and di-n-butyl tartrate in sodium tetraborate buffer. Ma et al. [141] described an *in situ* assembling of di-*n*-butyl-D-tartrate-boric acid complex which was used as a chiral selector. The higher sensitivity in chiral analysis of propranolol was achieved in connection with on-line sample preconcentration technique – field-amplified sample injection combined with water removal by electroosmotic low pump.

CEC- capillary electrochromatography has also become an important mode of CE for separation of enantiomers. It is a hybrid of CE and HPLC and combines the high efficacy of CE and high selectivity of HPLC. Chiral separation by CEC can be performed in wall-coated open tubular, packed and monolithic capillary column. Many chiral analyses have utilized chiral selectors based on macrocyclic antibiotics, mainly vancomycin [142, 143, 144, 145], teicoplanin [146], derivatives of cellulose and amylase [147, 148].

Fast excellent separation of propranolol was presented by Kumar and Park [149] using tris cellulose - (3,5-dimethylphenylcarbamate) modified zirconia monolithic column.

Glycidyl methacrylate –bonded β-cyclodextrine was introduced as a new chiral monomer in chiral separation of propranolol in CEC coupled to ESI-MS [150].

Indirect method resolution of propranolol enantiomers by CEC was conducted by Aturki et al. [151]. They used derivatization with (+)-1-(9-fluorenyl)ethyl chloroformate study. The prepared diastereoisomers were resolved on octadecylsilanized silica-gel based stationary phases.

Recently MCE-microchip electrophoresis has appeared to be suitable for separation of racemic compounds even in biological samples [152]. The miniaturization of analytical separation allows the consumption of samples and reagents be drastically reduced. Racemic propranolol was separated in the two enantiomers by a built MCE system coupled to a deep-UV fluorescence detection. The chiral separation was carried out in a fused-silica capillary containing S-α-CD and HS-α-CD [153].

Thin Layer Chromatography (TLC)

Thin layer chromatography is simple effective method for separation of enantiomers especially in commercial chiral pharmaceuticals, which can be done even in a small laboratory.

Direct enantiomeric resolution is achieved by preparing the TLC plate with chiral material or by adding a chiral selector to the mobile phase. Laboratory prepared chiral stationary phases on the base of cellulose trisphenylcarbamate derivatives [154, 155]: have been shown suitable for enantiomeric separation of some beta-blockers. The best resolution of racemic propranolol was obtained on cellulose tris(3,5-dimethylphenyl)carbamate.

Different amino acids impregnated into silica gel plates have been used for enantiomeric analysis of propranolol. These include: optically pure L-lysine (0.5 %) and L-arginine [156], *L*-glutamic and L-aspartic acids [157]. Beside L-aspartic acid also L-tartaric acid was used as a chiral selector [158]. Different combination of acetonitrile–methanol as mobile phases were found to be successful in resolving the enantiomers and spots were usually detected using iodine vapour.

Bushan and Tanwar used TLC plate impregnated by (-)erythromycin, pure L-tartaric acid, and (*R*)-mandelic acid for enantioresolution of atenolol and propranolol.

Some successful chiral resolution using a method of ligand–exchange processes TLC have been achieved using silica gel plates impregnated with Cu(II)-L-arginine complex [159]. Beta adrenolytics including propranolol were separated into their enantiomers by adopting different modes of loading/impregnating the Cu(II) complexes of L-proline, L-phenylalanine, L-histidine, *N,N*-dimethyl-L-phenylalanine, and L-tryptophan. Three different approaches based on ligand exchange mechanism were: a) using the Cu(II) –L-amino acid complex as chiral mobile phase additive, b) ascending development of plain silica gel plates in the solution of Cu(II) complex, and c) ascending development of plain silica gel plates in the solutions of amino acid and using a solution of Cu(II) acetate as a mobile phase additive. The detection limit was 0.18 μg for each enantiomer [159].

TLC enantioseparation of propranolol was also conducted on molecularly imprinted stationary phases. Several molecularly imprinted polymers were prepared using the enantiomer of (*R*)-propranolol as print molecule [160]. Suedee et al. [161] used molecularly imprinted polymers by α-agonists: (+)-ephedrine, (+)-pseudoephedrine (+)-norephedrine as chiral stationary phase.

Stereoselective Synthesis of Propranolol and Its Derivatives

Stereoselective synthesis involves chiral pool approach where the chiral centre is already built into one of the precursors and the resolution of racemic substrates mostly by kinetic way, when the individual enantiomers react at different speeds [162].

Two types of chemical catalysts are used for transformation of prochiral substances to enantiomerically enriched products in syntheses of propranolol or other aryloxyaminopropanolol derivatives.

Chiral Chemical Catalysis

Chiral chemical catalysis is based on the fact that the energy required for the formation of the complex of catalyst and one enantiomer is lower than that for the complex of the catalyst with the opposite enantiomer. Stereoselective catalysis using metal-ligand complexes is provided by coordination of enantiomeric ligands with a metal atom. The prochiral molecule of the substrate is bound to this complex. Second type of asymmetric chemical catalysis is using small chiral organic molecules without the presence of metals.

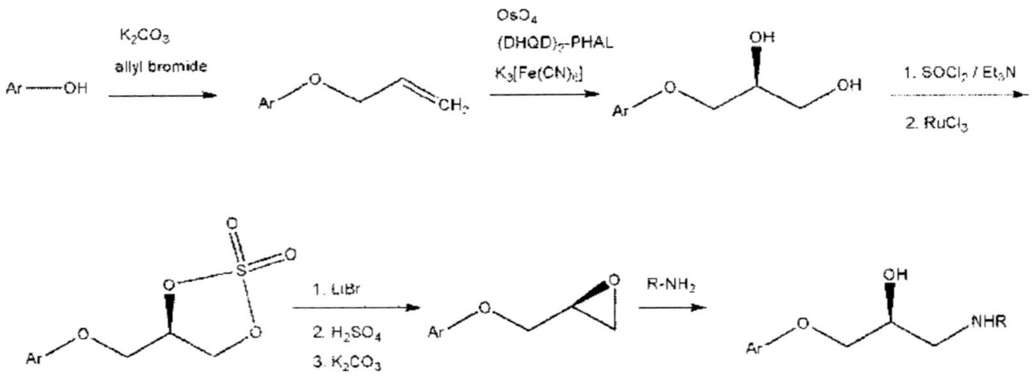

Figure 7. Asymmetric dihydroxylation of alylarylethers.

Optically inactive substrates are converted through a complex to optically active intermediates in several ways, such as asymmetric ring opening, asymmetric epoxidation, asymmetric dihydrogenation, regioselective substitution, metal-catalyzed kinetic resolution, hydrolytic kinetic resolution, kinetic resolution or ring opening reaction catalyzed by asymmetric nitroaldol reaction [162].

Chiral Catalysis Based on Metal-Ligand Complex

Asymmetric dihydroxylation of allyl aryl ethers catalyzed by osmium tetroxide was used for synthesis of seven (*S*)-3-arylpropane-1,2-diol intermediates in synthesis of propranolol and six other β-blockers **(Figure 7).**

The synthesis of propranolol started by the allylation of 1-naphthol with allyl bromide. The allylic ether was then subjected for osmium catalyzed Sharpless asymmetric dihydroxylation using (DHQD) 2 -PHAL (hydroquinidine 1,4-phthalazinediyl diether) as a chiral ligand and $K_3Fe(CN)_6/K_2CO_3$ as a co-oxidant to give the enantiomerically enriched diol. The diol reacted with thionyl chloride to form cyclic sulfite that was oxidized in the next step to cyclic sulfate by catalyzation of $RuCl_3$. The cyclic sulfate reacted with isopropylamine to afford propranolol. Low yield of this reaction was increased by using a three- step procedure with LiBr, H_2SO_4 and K_2CO_3/MeOH. Formed epoxide was then treated with isopropylamine in high overall yield and good enantiomeric excess (90 %) [163].

Hydrolytic kinetic resolution of terminal epoxides by using Jacobsen's catalyst is another possibility to obtain enantiomericaly pure propranolol and other aryloxyaminopropanol derivatives. Jacobsen's catalyst **(Figure 8)** presents a coordination compound of manganese (or cobalt, chromium) and salen – type ligand, *N,N'*-bis(3,5-di-*tert*-butylsalicylidene)-1,2-cyclohexanediamine, which can possess two conformations, (*R,R*) or (*S,S*).

The epoxide group of respective enantiomeric form of the substrate is hydrolyzed to a diol; an effective nucleophilic reagent for epoxide ring-opening reaction is a molecule of water **(Figure 9)**. Second enantiomer persists as the epoxide and can be used in the following condensation with isopropylamine to form propranolol. Resultant enantiomeric purity of the products is very high, in some cases up to 99 % [164, 165].

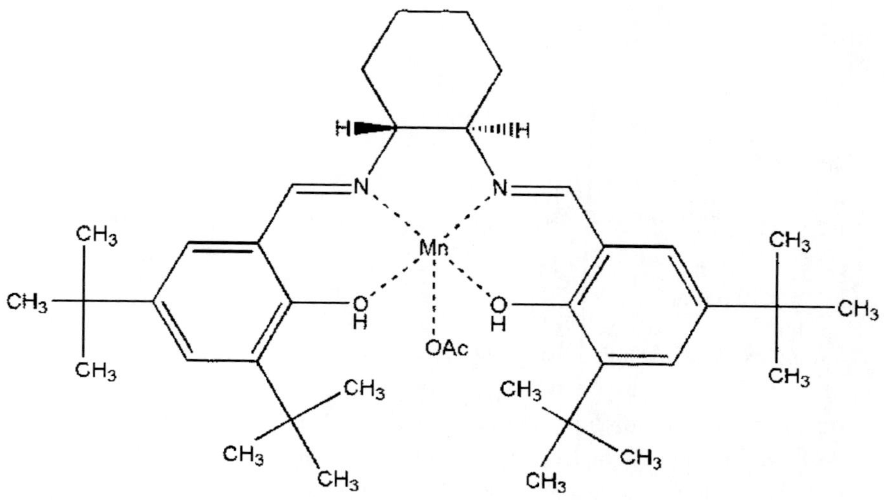

Figure 8. The structure of the Jacobsen's catalyst.

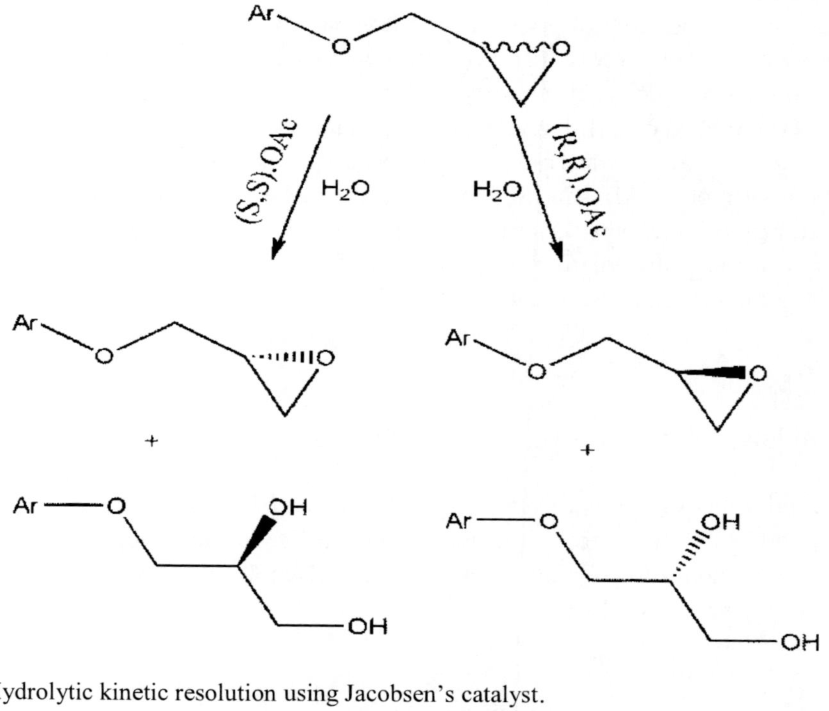

Figure 9. Hydrolytic kinetic resolution using Jacobsen's catalyst.

The method of hydrolytic kinetic resolution of racemic intermediates was also used by facile "one pot" synthesis of (*S*)-propranolol by using the catalysis of $Zn(NO_3)_2$ and L-tartaric acid. **(Figure 10)** [166]. Very similar method with small changes of reaction conditions was also published [167].

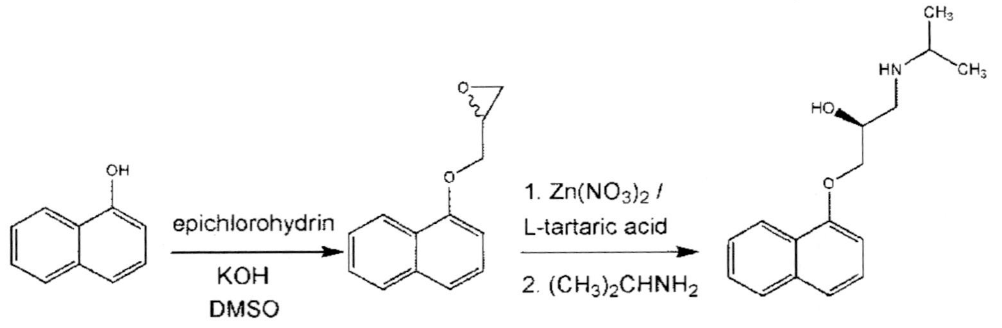

Figure 10. Hydrolytic kinetic resolution using $Zn(NO_3)_2$ and L-tartaric acid.

The stereoselective epoxidation of allylic alcohols (Sharpless epoxidation) is the next possible way to synthesize (*S*)- or (*R*)-epichlorohydrin or epoxy-intermediate of propranolol synthesis respectively. For this research, K. B. Sharpless was in 2001 awarded the Nobel Prize in chemistry. Allylic group undergoes oxidation to epoxide by using hydrogen peroxide as the oxidation reagent. Enantiomeric selection is provided by using titanium isopropoxide **(Figure 11)** [168].

(*S*)-propranolol is possible to obtain from racemate via stereoselective reduction of the aminoketone intermediate **(Figure 12)**. Prior to the synthesis the secondary amino group of propranolol was protected by di-*tert*-butylcarbonate (Boc_2O). Propranolol with protected aminogroup was oxidized by pyridinium chlorochromate (PCCl) to aminoketone. The ketonic group was then reduced by $NaBH_4$ in the presence of chloride of one of four examined divalent cations of metals (Mg, Ca, Sr, Ba). Divalent metal cation formed in the transition state a 5-membered cycle with ketone and ether oxygen **(Figure 13)** and increased the regioselectivity of the hydrogenation of the ketone. The enantiomeric excess decreased with increasing the ionic radius of metal cations, the highest was achieved using $MgCl_2$, 68.65 % ee [169].

Chiral Catalysis Based on Small Organic Molecules

The second type of stereoselective chemical catalysis involves pure organic low molecular weight substances not containing metal atoms in the process of bringing the asymmetric information into reaction products. One such molecule used as chiral catalyst in the synthesis of (*S*)-propranolol was L-proline.

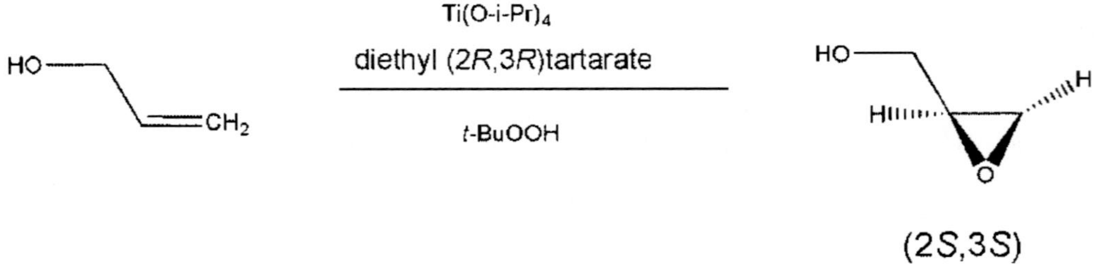

Figure 11. Sharpless epoxidation.

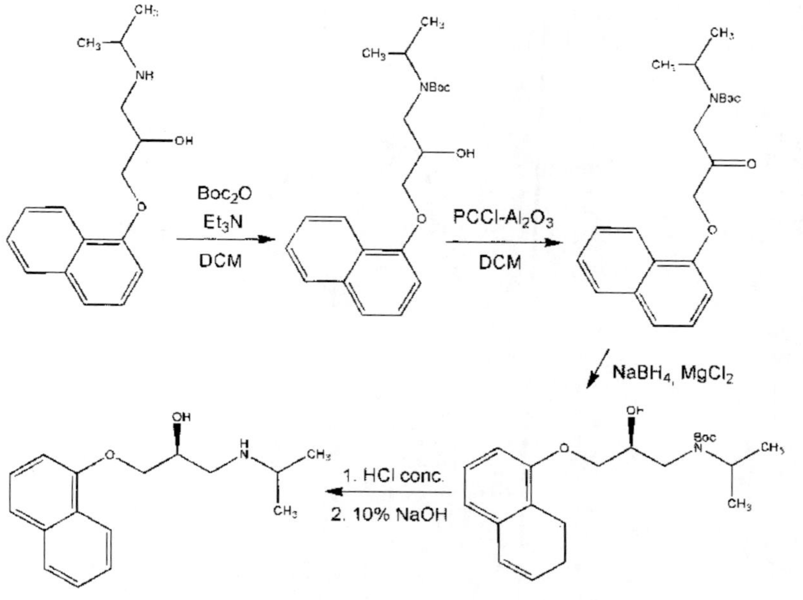

Figure 12. Stereoselective reduction of aminoketone intermediate.

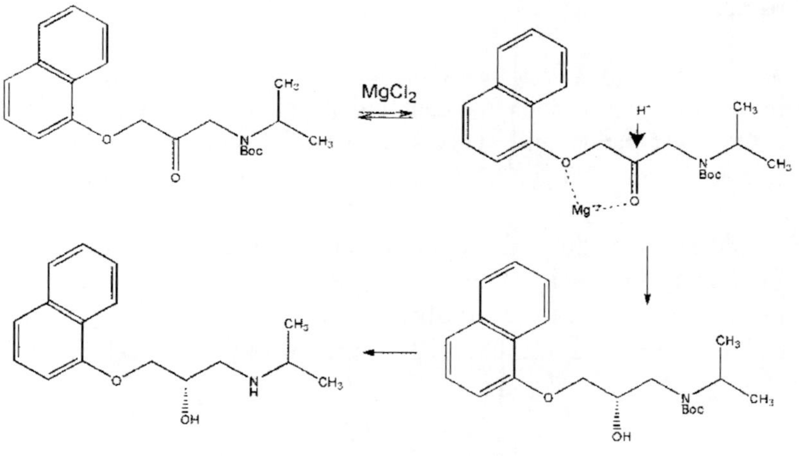

Figure 13. The transition state: 5-membered cycle of divalent metal cation with ketone and ether oxygen.

α-Naphthol, the input substrate was during the synthesis condensed with 3-bromopropanol. The 2-iodoxybenzoic acid (IBX) was used for the oxidation of the terminal alcohol group. The resulting aldehyde was converted into the chiral diol by using L-proline as a stereoselective catalyst in the presence of nitrosobenzene (PhNO); reduction was carried out using $NaBH_4$ in methanol followed by addition of Pd/C under a hydrogen atmosphere.

In the presence of triphenylphosphine (PPh_3) and diisopropyl azodicarboxylate (DIAD), the diol was transformed to the chiral epoxide, which was treated with isopropylamine resulting in (*S*)-propranolol **(Figure 14)**. The overall yield of the synthesis was 26 % and enantiomeric purity was 98 % ee [170].

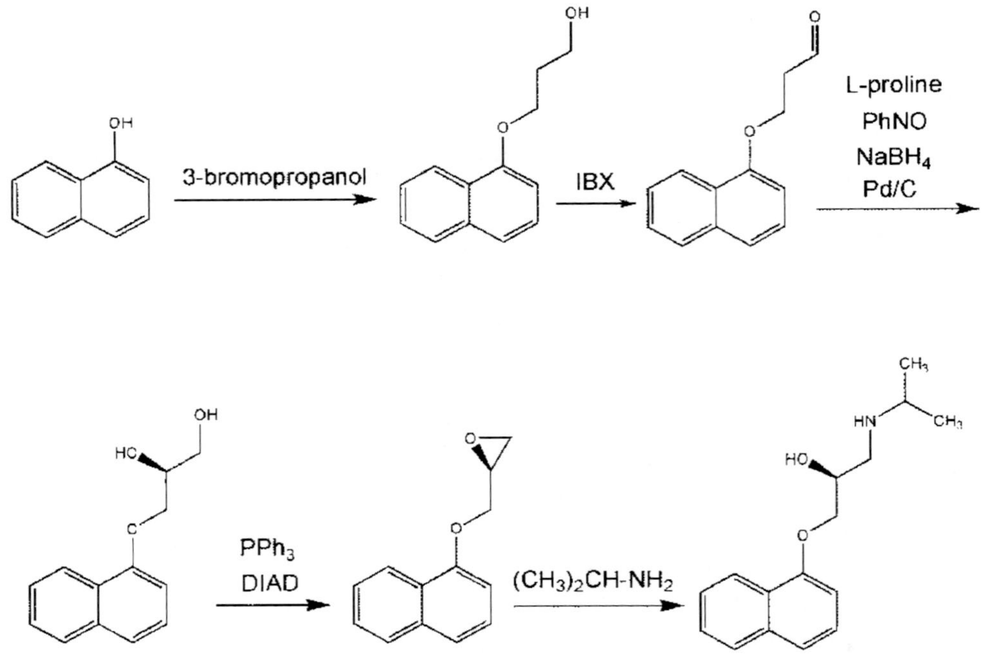

Figure 14. Chiral catalysis by L-proline.

Enantiomerically pure (*S*)-(−)-propranolol, was achieved also by synthesis starting from sorbitol. Via regioselective protection and coupling of α-naphthol, the key intermediate acetal was obtained. Its deprotection and successive oxidative degradation and a few simple conversion steps led to the formation of the enantiomer of propranolol with high optical purity [171].

Another synthesis starting from polyhydric alcohol was provided by the desymmetrization of glycerol with (*1R*)-(−)-10-camphorsulfonamide. Product of this reaction, an enantiopure spiroketal was successfully used for synthesis of both enantiomers of propranolol and naftopidil via the chiral 3-(1-naphthyloxy)propane-1,2-diol intermediate [172].

Chemo-Enzymatic Kinetic Resolution

Chemical catalyst in this process allows the flow of the reaction, but the resolution of enantiomers is provided by the enzyme, thereby allowing the formation of enantiomerically enriched intermediates. By enzymatic resolution the (*S*)-propranolol and (*S*)-alprenolol were prepared. Resolution of the racemic intermediate by the synthesis of propranolol was accomplished by means of enzyme-mediated enantioselective hydrolysis of the methyl ester intermediate in toluene and buffer **(Figure 15 on the left)**, or by enantioselective acylation of the hydroxyl group of the intermediate by vinyl acetate in the presence of lipase **(Figure 15 on the right)**.

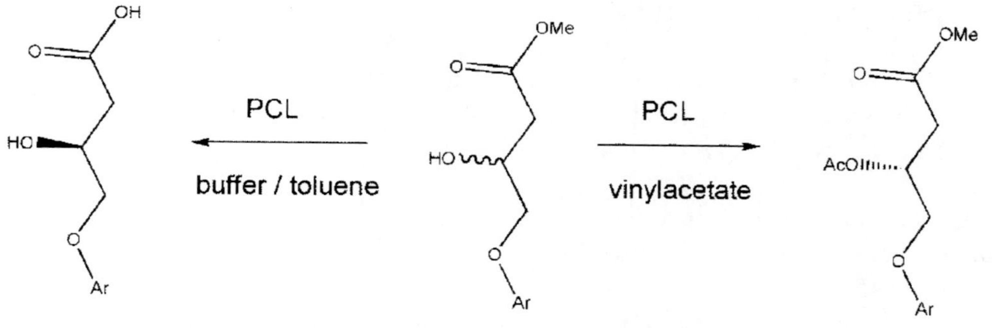

Figure 15. Chemo-enzymatic kinetic resolution.

Despite good enantiomeric yield the disadvantage of this approach is long reaction time. Yield and the lasting of the reaction depend on the type of the used enzyme. Higher enantiomeric efficiency and shorter reaction time were recorded using *Pseudomonas cepacia* lipase (PCL) compared to lipases isolated from *Porcine* pancreas, *Candida rugosa*, *Chromobacterium viscosum* and *Rhizomucor mieheia* [173].

The use of *P. cepacia* lipase immobilized on ceramic plates brought shorter reaction time required for the enantioselective transesterification of precursors of propranolol as compared with the free (non-immobilized) lipase [174].

Chemo-Enzymatic Dynamic Kinetic Resolution

Dynamic kinetic resolution combines enzymatic kinetic resolution of racemic precursors and in situ chemical racemization of the distomer. New onset racemate is again participating in the enzymatic kinetic resolution [175]. Prerequisite for successful dynamic kinetic resolution is mutual compatibility of kinetic resolution and racemization processes.

Dynamic kinetic resolution procedure was also applied on the azido-alcohol precursor of propranolol. The efficiency of the kinetic resolution was tested for various lipases; as an acyl donor the *p*-chlorophenylacetate (p-Cl-C_6H_4-OAc) was used. The highest activity has shown by using the lipase from *Pseudomonas cepacia*, the highest enantiomeric purity, however, has been reported with the use of lipase B from *Candida antarctica* (Novozyme 435, N-435). This enzyme has also been used in distinguishing the azido alcohols **(Figure 16)**. A ruthenium –based catalyst was the racemizing agents.. The chiral acetate of azido alcohol precursor was isolated in 71 % yield and enantiomeric purity of 86 % ee. By following "one-pot" procedure this intermediate was then converted in two steps to (*S*)-propranolol in almost pure enantiomeric form [176].

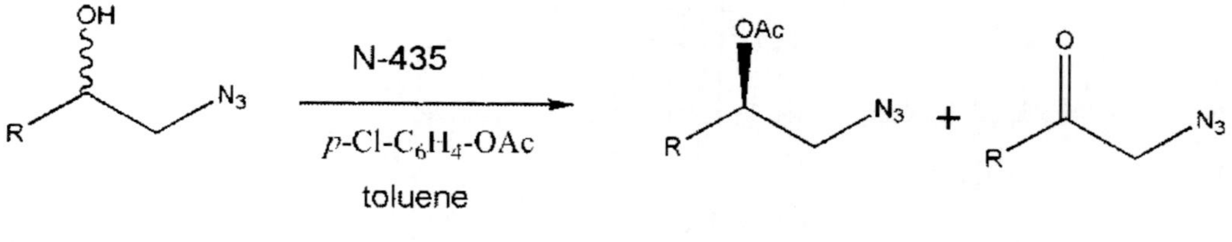

Figure 16. Dynamic kinetic resolution.

Resolution Using Cell Cultures

Cell cultures replace the actual enzymes in the reduction of racemic substrates. Broad spectrum of reductases, oxygenases or dehydrogenases contained in living cells expands possibilities of its use. The process may give higher yields in less time than enzymatic resolution.

Another advantage is cost savings on the isolating of the enzyme. Result of such resolution of enantiomers is affected by the type of substrate and the species of microorganism that has been used [162].

For the enantioselective reduction of prochiral ketones several microorganisms have been investigated. Beside the most commonly used baker's yeast, *Saccharomyces cerevisiae*, it was e. g. *Rhizopus arrhizus, Merulius tremellosus, Geotrichum candidum, Rhodococcus rubber*, or *Trichothecium* sp [177].

(*R*)- and (*S*)-enantiomers of propranolol were obtained in high optically pure form by the stereoselective hydrolysis of its acyl derivatives using whole cell preparations from *Trichosporon* sp., *Bacillus* sp. and pig liver. The results were compared with those obtained by using commercial lipases from *Mucor javanicus*, *Pseudomonas cepacia* and *Candida Antarctica* [178].

Chiral Pool Approach

Chiral pool approach to stereoselective synthesis of aryloxyaminopropanols involves the use of such substrates, wherein the specific chirality is already incorporated in its structure. Such syntheses are based mainly on natural substances such as D-mannitol, (*R*)-glyceraldehyde and L-ascorbic acid. The catalysts used in these syntheses do not distinguish the chirality of the substrate, only the total flow of the reaction is catalyzed.

Chiral propranolol precursors were synthesized from D-mannitol, which forms a cyclic acetal 1,2;5,6-di-*O*-diisopropylidenmanitol by reaction with acetone catalyzed by $ZnCl_2$. A higher yield was achieved by the reaction with 2,2-dimethoxypropane in DMSO catalyzed by *p*-toluenesulfonic acid. This intermediate was then oxidatively cleaved with sodium periodate or lead tetraacetate to two moles of (*R*)-2,3-*O*-izopropylidenglyceraldehyde. Chiral precursor (*S*)-2,3-*O*-isopropylidene was prepared by reduction of this intermediate with $NaBH_4$ **(Figure 17)** [179].

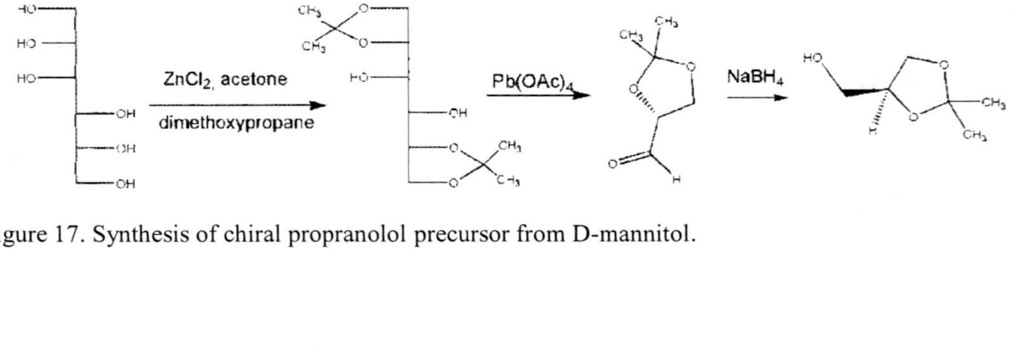

Figure 17. Synthesis of chiral propranolol precursor from D-mannitol.

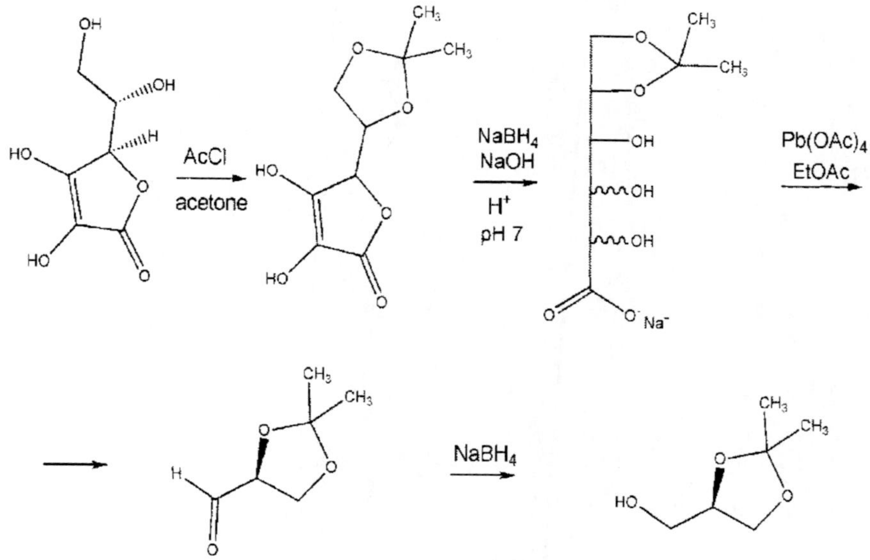

Figure 18. Synthesis of chiral propranolol precursor from **L**-ascorbic acid.

By synthesis starting from L-ascorbic acid the opposite enantiomeric form of the precursor, (*R*)-2,3-*O*-isopropylidene, can be produced. L-ascorbic acid treated with acetyl chloride in acetone yielding 5,6-*O*-isopropylidene-L-ascorbic acid, which after reduction with $NaBH_4$ followed by hydrolysis using NaOH gave an intermediate that was cleaved by lead tetraacetate to gave (*R*)-2,3-*O*-izopropylideneglyceraldehyde. Reduction of this intermediate with $NaBH_4$ resulted in final chiral precursor (*R*)-2,3-*O*-isopropylidene **(Figure 18)** [180].

These intermediates could be used in the synthesis of aryloxyaminopropanols as 2,3-O-isopropylideneglyceroltosylates which were prepared by reaction with *p*-toluensulphochloride in pyridine [179]. Very similar synthesis of (*S*)-propranolol from D-mannitol with a small changes of reagent agents was also published [181].

D-mannitol was the starting material also for the asymmetric synthesis of (*S*)-propranolol via (*S*)-5-hydroxymethyl-3-isopropyl-2-oxazolidinone which was a result of enzymatic resolution of this low carbon sugar alcohol. (*S*)-propranolol was produced in overall yield 65 % and enantiomeric purity 99 % ee [182].

Stereoselective Extraction

To distinguish the enantiomers of β-blockers two extraction methods have been developed. In both, adding of the chiral selector in one of the phases is a must. Extraction by two mutually immiscible liquids may be biphasic, when the chiral selector is bound to one enantiomer and allowed the other to redistribute to the second phase, or membrane-type, wherein the selector is fixed on a membrane, thereby allowing cross-membrane moving only for one enantiomer.

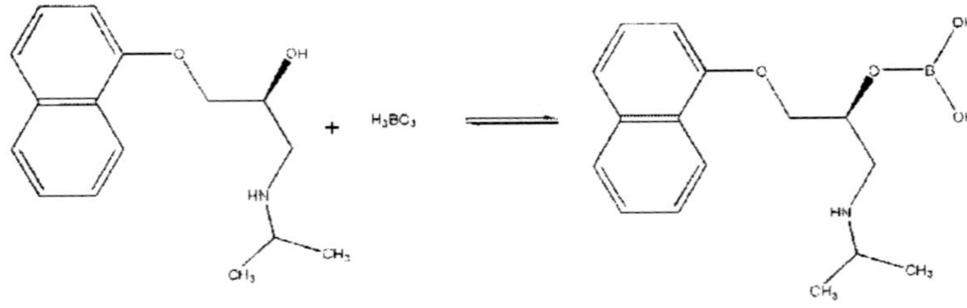

(*R*)-propranolol (*R*)-propranolol borate ester

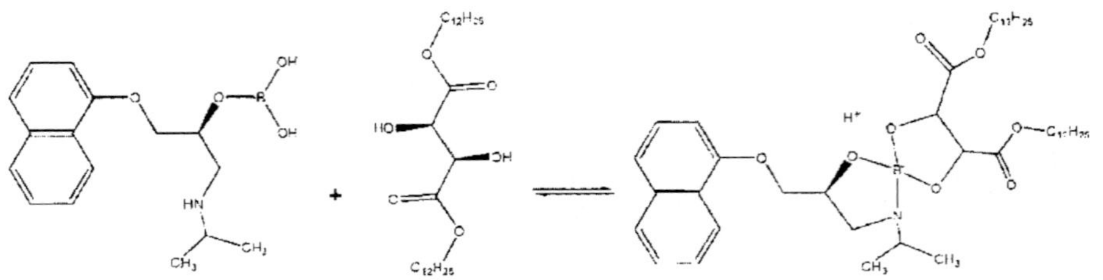

(*R*)-di-*n*-dodecyltartarate (*R*)-propranolol-borate-(*R*)-tartarate complex

Figure 19. Stereoselective extraction – synthesis of the complex of propranolol with boric acid and (R)- and (S)-di-n-dodecyltartrate.

The racemic mixture of propranolol was partitioned in a two phase system of chloroform / water by using a complex with boric acid and (*R*)- and (*S*)-di-*n*-dodecyltartrate in the enantiomeric excess of 1.0 to 9.3 % **(Figure 19).** Enantioseparation was affected by the pH of the aqueous phase, the best results were obtained with acetate buffer at pH 5.2 [183].

The second method of extraction published by the same team of authors is based on the presence of the same chiral selector fixed on a ceramic membrane. (*S*)-propranolol remained in the aqueous phase and the (*R*)-isomer was transported into chloroform. Process has achieved enantiomeric purity of 40 % ee [184].

Crystallization of Salts with Optically Active Acids

Optically active analogues of propranolol were prepared by resolution with *p*-(−)ditolyltartaric acid. After recrystallization of the precipitated (−)-salt from isopropyl alcohol the (*S*)-(−)-enantiomer was isolated as the hydrochloride in good enantiomeric excess. Using of dibenzoyltartaric acid concluded to unsuccessful resolution [185].

Some other optically active acids, such as (+)-malic acid, (*2R,3R*)-(+)-tartaric acid or (*R*)-(−)-mandelic acid are also useful for resolution of such enantiomers of aryloxyaminopropanol β-blockers [179].

Conclusion

Propranolol (1-(1-naphthyloxy)-3-(isopropylamino)propan-2-ol.HCl) is the most well-known nonselective adrenergic antagonist (β_1, β_2 - blocker), a beta-adrenergic blocker used therapeutically in the treatment of angina pectoris and hypertension as well as in the prevention of hyperthyroidism, migraine or anxiety. Propranolol is based on an aryloxyaminopropanol scaffold (as are its derivatives), and is synthesized in two steps from naphthalen-1-ol by reaction with chloromethyloxirane and subsequent treatment with isopropylamine. Propranolol is used as a racemic salt with hydrochloric acid in therapeutic practice.

Propranolol possess a stereogenic centre and can form different (*R*)-(+) and (*S*)-(−)-enantiomers. These enantiomers exhibit marked differences in biological activities such as their pharmacodynamics, pharmacokinetics, toxicology and metabolism.

The major bioactive enantiomer – the eutomer – is (*S*)-(−)-propranolol, whose antiadrenergic effect is many times stronger than that of its less active distomer, the (*R*)-(+)-enantiomer, which manifests various adverse effects. (*R)*-(+)-propranolol is known to act as a contraceptive; racemic form of propranolol and unlike the (*S*)-(−)-enantiomer, inhibits the conversion of thyroxin to triiodothyronine. Differences in the pharmacokinetics of propranolol enantiomers were observed in the drug's distribution (stereospecifically bound to plasma proteins) and elimination (the stereospecificity of liver enzymes). Stereoselective binding to the β-adrenoceptor induces differences in its pharmacodynamics.

Various methods are used for the chiral separation of propranolol enantiomers at both the analytical and preparative scale. The most widely used technique for the separation and quantification of enantiomers is enantioselective high-performance liquid chromatography. The chiral separation of propranolol and its analogues can be performed using different chiral stationary phases based on proteins, cyclodextrins, modified polysaccharides (cellulose, amylose), or macrocyclic antibiotics (vancomycin, teicoplanin). The enantioseparation of propranolol by gas chromatography requires a chiral derivatizing agent (N-heptafluorobutyryl anhydride, *N,O*-bis(trimethylsilyl)trifluoroacetamide, trifluoroacetic anhydride, *N*-trifluoracetyl-(*S*)-(−)-prolylchloride), which converts enantiomers into diastereoisomers. A similar mechanism for the enantioseparation of propranolol is used in thin-layer chromatography. The TLC silica gel plates are impregnated with L-aspartic acid or L-glutamic acid as the chiral selector. Another reliable technique for the chiral separation of propranolol is capillary electrophoresis. Propranolol enantiomers separated via this method are resolved by the addition of modified cyclodextrin as a chiral selector (hydroxypropyl beta-CD, dimethyl beta-CD, carboxymethyl beta-CD). Cellulose derivatives or human serum albumin can also be used as chiral selectors for capillary electrophoresis.

Single (*R*)-(+) and (*S*)-(−)-enantiomers with different levels of enantiomeric purity can be obtained using several methods of stereoselective synthesis. The stereoselective synthesis of propranolol enantiomers can be catalysed by complexes of ligands and various metals: e. g., catalysis of the asymmetric dihydroxylation of allyl aryl ethers with OsO_4, catalysis of the hydrolytic kinetic resolution of epoxides with the Jacobsen catalyst or with $Zn(NO_3)_2$ and L-tartaric acid, and catalysis of the Sharpless asymmetric oxidation or stereoselective reduction of the ketone intermediate in the presence of a divalent metal cation. Low-molecular organic compounds such as L-proline can be used as the chiral catalysts for the preparation of single enantiomers of propranolol. Chemo-enzymatic routes could be also used for this purpose, with the chemical catalyst enabling reaction flow and the enzyme, typically a lipase or whole yeast cells, providing for the stereoselectivity of the reaction. The stereoselective synthesis of propranolol may also be achieved using chiral pool methods, where the synthesis starts from enantiomerically pure substrates. D-mannitol and L-ascorbic acid are described in the literature as suitable substrates.

The resolution of propranolol racemate at preparative scale was achieved using (+)-*O,O′*-di-p-toluoyl-*(R,R)*-tartaric acid and (–)-*O,O′*-di-p-toluoyl-(*S,S*)-tartaric acid. Propranolol stereoisomers were separated via a multi-step recrystallization of its salts with di-(p-toluoyl) tartaric acid.

Stereoselective extraction in a biphasic system using a chiral selector in one of the phases or fixed to a membrane is also described in this chapter.

References

[1] Akbar, S; Alorainy, MS. The current status of beta blockers' use in the management of hypertension. *Saudi Med. J.*, 2014, 35, p. 1307-1317.

[2] Lechat, P. Clinical pharmacology of beta-blockers in cardiology: trial results and clinical applications. *Hot Topics in Cardiology*, 2008, 10, p. 7–44.

[3] Lin, HW; Phan, K; Lin, SJ. Trends in off-label β-blocker use: a secondary data analysis. *Clin. Ther.*, 2006, 28, p. 1736-1746.

[4] Baker, JG; Hill, SJ; Summera, RJ. Evolution of β-blocker: from anti-anginal drugs to ligand-directed signalling. *Trends. Pharmacol.*, *Sci.* 2011, 32 (4), p. 227-234.

[5] Borthne, A. The treatment of glaucoma with propranolol (Inderal). A clinical trial. *Acta Ophthalmo*l., (Copenh) 1976, 54 (3), p. 291-300.

[6] Brunet, A; Orr, SP; Tremblay, J; Robertson, K; Nader, K; Pitman, RK. Effect of post-retrieval propranolol on psychophysiologic responding during subsequent script-driven traumatic imagery in post-traumatic stress disorder. *J. Psychiatr. Res.*, 2008, 42, p. 503-506.

[7] Hepp, Z; Bloudek, L; Varon, SF. Systematic review of migraine prophylaxis adherence and persistence. *J. Manag. Care Pharm.*, 2014, 20, p. 22-33.

[8] Benvenisti, H; Ben-Sira, L; Constantini, S; Roth, J. Giant cranial and cerebellar hemangioma treated with propranolol. *Childs Nerv. Syst.*, 2014, in press.

[9] Stapleton, MP. Sir James Black and propranolol. The role of the basic sciences in the history of cardiovascular pharmacology. *Tex. Heart Inst., J.* 1997, 24, p. 336-342.

[10] Black, JW; Crowther, AF; Shanks, RG; Smith, LH; Dornhorst, AC., A new adrenergic betareceptor antagonist. *Lancet*, 1964, 283, p. 1080-1081.

[11] Pchelka, BK; Loupy, A; Petit, A. Improvement and simplification of synthesis of 3-aryloxy-1,2-epoxypropanes using solvent-free conditions and microwave irradiations. Relation with medium effects and reaction mechanism. *Tetrahedron*, 2006, 62, p. 10968-10979.

[12] Crowther, AF; Smith, LH. *Propranolol synthesis.*, 1967, U.S. Patent 3, 337, 628.

[13] Čižmáriková, R; Chudáčiková, S; Valentová, J; Némethy, A. Synthesis and enantioseparation of derivatives of propranolol. *Acta Fac. Pharm. Univ. Comen.*, 2012, 59, p. 5-13.

[14] Inkum, R; Teerawutgulrag, A; Puangsombat, P; Rakariyatham, N., An alternative synthesis of (±)-propranolol and (±) atenolol. *Maejo. Inj. J. Sci. Technol.*, 2012, 3 (6), p. 372-378.

[15] Kureshy, RI; Ahmad, I; Pathak, K; Khan, NH; Abdi, SHR; Bajaj, HC; Suresh, E. Solvent-free microwave synthesis of aryloxypropanolamine by ring opening of aryloxy epoxides. Research Letters in Organic Chemistry 2009, 10, Article ID 109717, 5 pages.

[16] Jovanovic, S; Vico-Stefanovic, M; Ugljesic-Kilibarda, D; Popadic, D. Catalyst in the alkylation reaction of 1.naphtol with epichlorohydrin. *J. Serb. Chem. Soc.*, 2006, 71 (8-9), p. 867-877.

[17] www.drugs.com. [Online] 7. 12. 2014. http://www.drugs.com/pro/ propranolol.html.

[18] Wang, X; Wang, XJ; Ching, CB. Solubility metastable zone width, and racemic characterization of propranolol hydrochloride. *Chirality*, 2002, 14, p. 318-324.

[19] Howe, R; Shanks, RG. Optical isomers of propranolol. *Nature*, 1966, 210, p. 1336-1338.

[20] Nguyen, LA; He, H; Pham-Huy, Ch. Chiral Drugs: An Overview. *Int. J. Biomed. Sci.*, 2006, 2, p. 85-100.

[21] Čižmáriková, R. β-Adrenergic receptor blockers – a group of chiral drugs: different effect of each enantiomer. *Čes. Slov. Farm.*, 2002, 51, p. 121-128 (in slovak).

[22] Cahn, RS; Ingold, CK; Prelog, V. The specification of asymmetric configuration in organic chemistry. *Experientia*, 1956, 3, p. 81-124.

[23] Patil, PN; Lapidus, JB. Stereoisomerism in adrenergic drug. *Ergebnisse der physiologie, biologischen Chemie and experimentellen Pharmakologie*, 1972, 66, p. 213-260.

[24] Soriano-Ursúa, MA; Trujillo-Ferrara, JG; Correa-Basurto, J. Homology modeling and flex-ligand docking studies on guinea pig β2 adrenoceptor: structural and experimental similarities/ differences with human β2. *J. Mol. Model.*, 2009, 15, p. 1203-1211.

[25] Polakovičová, M; Čižmáriková, R. Molecular docking study on the binding mode of cardioselective phenoxyaminopropanol blocker into β-adrenergic receptor subtypes. *Acta Fac. Pharm. Univ. Comen.*, 2012, 59, p. 44-52.

[26] Kuipers, W; Link, R; Standaar, PJ; Stoit, AR; Van Wijngaarden, I; Leurs, R; Ijzerman, AP. Study of the interaction between aryloxypropanolamines and Asn386 in helix VII of the human 5-hydroxytryptamine1A receptor. *Mol. Pharmacol.*, 1997, 51, p. 889-896.

[27] Hutt, AJ; O´Grady, J. Drug chirality: a consideration of the significance of the stereochemistry of antimicrobial agents. *J. Antimicrob. Chemother.*, 1996, 37, p. 7-32.

[28] Lemke, TL; Williams, DA; Roche, VF; Zito, SW. *Foye's principles of Medicinal Chemistry (6 ed.).* Philadelphia: Lippincott Williams & Wilkins, 2008. ISBN 978-0-7817-6879-5.

[29] Stoschitzky, K; Lindner, W; Kiowski, W. Stereoselective vascular effects of the (*R*)- and (*S*)-enantiomers of propranolol and atenolol. *J. Cardiovasc. Pharmacol.*, 1995, 25, p. 268-272.

[30] Barrett, AM; Cullum, VA. The biological properties of the optical isomers of propranolol and their effect on cardiac arrhythmias. *Br. J. Pharmacol.*, 1968, 34, p. 43-55.

[31] Belpaire, FM; Wynant, P; Van Trappen, P; Dhont, M; Vestraete, A; Bogaert, MG. Protein binding of propranolol and verapamil enantiomers in maternal and foetal serum. *Br. J. Clin. Pharmacol.*, 1995, 39, p. 190-193.

[32] Mehvar, R; Brocks, DR. Stereospecific pharmacokinetics and pharmacodynamic of beta-adrenergic blockers in humans. *J. Pharm. Pharmaceut. Sci.*, 2001, 4, p. 185-200.

[33] Takahashi, H; Ogata, H; Kanno, S; Takeuchi, H. Plasma protein binding of propranolol enantiomers as major determinant of their stereoselective tissue distribution in rats. *J. Pharmacol. Exp. Ther.*, 1990, 252, p. 272-278.

[34] Marathe, PH; Shen, DD; Nelson, WL. Metabolic kinetics of pseudoracemic propranolol in human liver microsomes. Enantioselectivity and quinidine inhibition. *Drug Metab. Dispos.*, 1994, 22, p. 237-247.

[35] Masubuchi,Y; Hosokawa, S; Horie, T; Suzuki, T; Ohmori, S; Kitada, M; Narimatsu, S. Cytochrome P450 isozymes involved in propranolol metabolism in human liver microsomes. The role of CYP2D6 as ring-hydroxylase and CYP1A2 as N-desisopropylase. *Drug Metab. Dispos.*, 1994, 22 , p. 909-915.

[36] Walle, T; Webb, JG; Bagwell, EE; Walle, UK; Daniell, HB; Gaffney, TE. Stereoselective delivery and actions of beta receptor antagonists. *Biochem. Pharmacol.*, 1988, 37, p. 115-124.

[37] Walle, T. Stereoselectivity of the in vivo disposition and metabolism of propranolol in dog and man using deuterium-labeled pseudoracemates. *Drug Metab. Dispos.*, 1985, 13, p. 279-282.

[38] Bode, W; Toest, AE; Stolker, AA; van Ginkel, LA; Groen, K; Wermer, J; de Wildt, DJ. Toxicokinetic of a single intravenous dose of rac-propranolol versus optically pure propranolol in the rat. *Chirality*, 1995, 7, 626-631.

[39] Toet, AE; van de Kuil, A; Vleeming, W; Wemer, J; Bode, W; Meulenbelt, J; de Wildt, DJ. Toxic doses of rac-, (-)-(*S*)- and (+)-(*R*)-propranolol in rats and rabbits. *Chirality*, 1996, 8, 411-417.

[40] Stanley, JK; Ramirez, AJ; Mottaleb, M; Chambliss, CK; Brooks, BW. Enantiospecific toxicity of the beta-blocker propranolol to Daphnia magna and Pimephales promelas. *Environ. Toxicol. Chem.*, 2006, 25, 1780-1786.

[41] Wang, DW; Mistry, AM; Kahlig, KM; Kearney, JA; Xiang, J; George, AL. Jr. Propranolol blocks cardiac and neuronal voltage-gated sodium channels. *Front Pharmacol.*, 2010, 1 (1), p. 144.

[42] Srivastava, S; Coutinho, E. Adrenergic antagonist propranolol as a novel, effective spermicide: an NMR study. *J. Pharm. Sci. Pharmacol.*, 2010, 2, 196-201.

[43] Stoschitzky, K; Lindner, W; Egginger, G; Brunner, F; Obermayer-Pietsch, B; Passath, A; Klein, W. Racemic (*R*,*S*)-propranolol versus half-dosed optically pure (*S*)-propranolol in humans at steady state: Hemodynamic effects, plasma concentrations, and influence on thyroid hormone levels. *Clin. Pharmacol. Ther.*, 1992, 51, 445-453.

[44] Suedee, R; Brain, KR; Heard, Ch. M. Differential permeation of propranolol enantiomers across human skin in vitro from formulation containing an enantioselective excipient. *Chirality*, 1999, 11, 680-683.

[45] Fischer, W. Anticonvulsant profile and mechanism of action of propranolol and its two enantiomers. *Seizure*, 2002, 11, 285-302.

[46] Forssén, P; Arnell, R; Kaspereit, M; Seidel-Morgenstern, A; Fornstedt, T. Effects of a strongly adsorbed additive on process performance in chiral preparative chromatography. *J. Chromatogr.*, *A* 2008, 1212, 89-97.

[47] Torul, H; Tamer, U. Determination of enantiomers of atenolol and propranolol in pharmaceutical formulations by HPLC. *J. AOAC Int.*, 2011, 94, 833-888.

[48] Pham-Huy, C; Sahui-Gnassi, A; Saada, V; Gramond, JP; Galons, H; Ellouk-Achard, S; Levresse, V; Fompeydie, D; Claude, JR. Microassay of propranolol enantiomers and

conjugates in human plasma and urine by high-performance liquid chromatography after chiral derivatization for pharmacokinetic study. *J. Pharm. Biomed. Anal.*, 1994, 12, 1189-1198.

[49] Wu, ST; Chang, YP; Gee, WL; Benet, LZ; Lin, ET. Stereoselective high-performance liquid chromatography determination of propranolol and 4-hydroxypropranolol in human plasma after pre-column derivatization. *J. Chromatogr. B Biomed. Sci. Appl.*, 1997, 692, 133-40.

[50] Morante-Zarcero, S; Sierra, I. Comparative HPLC methods for β-blockers separation using different types of chiral stationary phases in normal phase and polar organic phase elution modes. Analysis of propranolol enantiomers in natural waters. *J. Pharm. Biomed. Anal.*, 2012, 62, 33-41.

[51] Gübitz, G; Schmid, MG. Chiral separation principles. *In. Chiral separations.*, Totowa, New Jersey: Humana Press, 2004, 1-28.

[52] Marko, V. *Determination of Beta-Blockers in Biological Material: Evaluation of Analytical Methods in Biological Systems.* Amsterdam: Elsevier Science Publishers B. V., 1989. ISBN 0-444-87305-8.

[53] Dyas, AM. The chiral chromatographic separation of β-adrenoceptor blocking drugs. *J. Pharmacol. Biomed. Anal.*, 1992, 10, 383-404.

[54] Čižmáriková, R; Valentová, J; Hutt, JA. Beta-adrenergic blockers- a group of chiral drugs: enantioseparation in the group of β-blockers. *Čes. Slov. Farm.*, 2004, 53, 9-17. (in slovak).

[55] Kačeriaková, D; Špánik, I. Utilization of cyclodextrins in gas chromatography: preparation of capillary columns with cyclodextrin stationary phases. *Chem. Listy*, 2014, 108, 462-469. (in slovak).

[56] Dönnecke, J; Paul, C; König, WA; Svensson, LA; Gyllenhaal, O; Vessman, J. Immobilization of heptakis 6-*O*-*terc*-butyldimethylsilyl-2,3-di-*O*-methyl)-β-cyclodextrin for capillary gas chromatography and SFC and microliquid chromatography. *J. Microcolumn, Sep.* 1996, 8, 495-505.

[57] Abe, I; Nishiyama, T; Nakahara, T; Frank, H. Gas chromatographic enantiomer separation of pharmaceuticals on capillary columns coated with novel chiral polysiloxanes. *J. Chromatogr., A* 1995, 694, 237-243.

[58] König, WA; Ernst, K. Improved gas chromatographic enantiomer separation of pharmaceutically relevant amino alcohols as oxazolidinones. *J. Chromatogr.*, 1984, 294, 423-426.

[59] Thomson, JA; Holtzman, JL; Tsuru, M; Lerman, Ch. L; Holtzman, JL. Procedure for the chiral derivatization and chromatographic resolution of (*R*)- and (*S*) –propranolol. *J. Chromatogr.*, 1982, 238, 470-475.

[60] Saelens, DA; Walle, T; Provitera, PJ. Quantitative determination of propranolol glycol and N-desisopropylpropranolol in brain tissue by electron capture gas chromatography. *J. Chromatogr.*, 1976, 123, 185-192.

[61] Caccia, S; Guiso, G; Ballabio, M; De ponte, P. Simultaneous determination of the propranolol enantiomers in biological samples by gas-liquid chromatography. *J. Chromatogr.*, 1979, 172, 457-462.

[62] Caccia, S; Chiabrando, C; De-Ponte, P; Fanelli, R. Separation of beta adrenoceptor antagonist enantiomers by high resolution capillary gas chromatography. *J. Chromatogr., Sci.* 1979, 16, 543-546.

[63] Bojarski, J. Stereoselective chromatography of cardiovascular drugs: an update. *J. Biochem. Biophys. Methods*. 2002, 54, 197-220.

[64] Shao, G; Goto, J; Nambara, T. Separation and Determination of Propranolol Enantiomers in Plasma by High-Performance Liquid Chromatography with Fluorescence Detection. *J. Liq. Chromatogr.*, 1991, 14, 753-763.

[65] Laganière, S; Kwong, E; Shen, DD. Stereoselective high-performance liquid chromatographic assay for propranolol enantiomers in serum. *J. Chromatogr.*, 1989, 488, 407-416.

[66] Roux, A; Blanchot, G; Baglin, A; Flouvat, B. Liquid chromatographic analysis of propranolol enantiomers in human blood using precolumn derivatization with (+)-1-(9-fluorenyl)ethyl chloroformate. *J. Chromatogr.*, 1991, 570, 453-461.

[67] Prakash, C; Koshakji, RP; Wood, AJ; Blair, IA. Simultaneous determination of propranolol enantiomers in plasma by high-performance liquid chromatography with fluorescence detection. *J. Pharm. Sci.*, 1989, 78, 771-775.

[68] Pflugmann, G; Spahn, H; Mutschler, E. Rapid determination of the enantiomers of metoprolol, oxprenolol and propranolol in urine. *J. Chromatogr.*, 1987, 416, 331-339.

[69] Lindner, W; Rath, M; Stoschitzky, K; Uray, G. Enantioselective drug monitoring of (*R*)- and (*S*)- propranolol in human plasma via derivatization with optically active (*R*,*R*)-*O*,*O*-diacetyl tartaric acid anhydride. *J. Chromatogr.*, 1989, 487, 375-383.

[70] Kleidernigg, OP; Lindner, W. Synthesis of new stable aliphatic isocyanate-based chiral derivatizing agent and application to indirect separation of chiral amino and thio compounds. *Chromatographia.*, 1997, 44, 465-472.

[71] Péter, M; Gyéresi, A; Fülöp, F. Liquid chromatographic enantioseparation of beta-blocking agents with (*1R*,*2R*)-1,3-diacetoxy-1-(4-nitrophenyl)-2-propyl isothiocyanate as chiral derivatizing agent. *J. Chromatogr., A.* 2001, 910, 247-253.

[72] Toyo'oka, T; Toriumi, M. Enantioseparation of beta-blockers labelled with a chiral fluorescent reagent, *R* (-)-DBD-PyNCS, by reversed-phase liquid chromatography. *J. Pharm. Biomed. Anal.*, 1997, 15, 1467-1476.

[73] Toyo'oka, T; Jin, D; Tomoi, N; Oe ,T; Hiranuma, H. (*R*)-(-)-4-(3-isothiocyanatopyrrolidin-1-yl)-7-(*N*,*N*-dimethylaminosulfonyl)-2,1,3-benzoxadiazole, a fluorescent chiral tagging reagent: sensitive resolution of chiral amines and amino acids by reversed-phase liquid chromatography. *Biomed. Chromatogr.*, 2001, 15, 56-67.

[74] Bhushan, R; Tanwar, S. Reversed-phase high-performance liquid chromatographic enantioresolution of six beta-blockers using dinitrophenyl-L-Pro-*N*-hydroxysuccinimide ester, *N*-succinimidyl-(*S*)-2-(6-methoxynaphth-2-yl) propionate and twelve variants of Sanger's reagent as chiral derivatizing reagents. *Biomed. Chromatogr.*, 2009, 23, 1291-1299.

[75] Bhushan, R; Dixit, S. Enantioresolution of five β-blockers by reversed-phase high-performance liquid chromatography using fifteen chiral derivatizing reagents having amino acids or their amides as chiral auxiliaries on a cyanuric chloride platform. *Biomed. Chromatogr.*, 2012, 26, 239-246.

[76] Yu, L; Luan. L; Shao, Q; Zeng, S. Direct determination of (*S*)-(-)- and (*R*)-(+)-propranolol glucuronide in rat hepatic microsomes by RP-HPLC. *Biomed. Chromatogr.*, 2004, 18, 833-837.

[77] Younes, AA; Mangelings, D; Van der Heyden, Y. Chiral separations in normal phase liquid chromatography: enantioselectivity of recently commercialized polysaccharide-

based selectors. Part I: enantioselectivity under generic screening conditions. *J. Pharm. Biomed. Anal.*, 2011, 55, 414-423.

[78] Enquist, M; Hermansson, J. Separation of the enantiomers of beta-receptor blocking agents and other cationic drugs using a CHIRAL-AGP column. Binding properties and characterization of immobilized alpha 1-acid glycoprotein. *J. Chromatogr.*, 1990, 519, 285-298.

[79] Matsunaga, H; Haginaka, J. Separation of enantiomers on chiral stationary phase based on chicken α-acid glycoprotein: effect of silica particle diameters on column performance. *J. Chromatogr., A.* 2014, 1363, 96-100.

[80] Matchett, MW; Branch, SK; Jefferies, TM. Polar organic chiral separation of propranolol and analogues using a β-cyclodextrin bonded stationary phase. *Chirality*, 1996, 8, 126-130.

[81] Pham-Huy, C; Radenen, B; Sahui-Gnassi, A; Claude, JR. High-performance liquid chromatographic determination of (*S*)- and (*R*)-propranolol in human plasma and urine with a chiral beta-cyclodextrin bonded phase. *J. Chromatogr. B Biomed. Appl.*, 1995, 665, 125-132.

[82] Petersen, PV; Ekelund, J; Olsen, L; Ovesen, SV. Chiral separations of β-blocking drug substances using the Pirkle-type alpha-Burke 1 chiral stationary phase. *J. Chromatogr. A*, 1997, 757, 65-71.

[83] Singh, AK; Kedor-Hackmann, Erika RM; Santoro, Maria Inês RM. Enantiomeric separation and quantitative determination of propranolol enantiomers in pharmaceutical preparations by chiral liquid chromatography. *Rev. Bras. Cienc. Farm*,. 2004, 40, 301-304.

[84] Čižmáriková, R; Račanská, E; Hroboňová, K; Lehotay, J; Aghová, Z; Halešová, D. Synthesis, pharmacological activity and chromatographic separation of some novel potential β-blockers of the aryloxyaminopropanol type. *Pharmazie.*, 2003, 58, 237-241.

[85] Kafková, B; Bosáková, Z; Tesarová, E; Coufal, P. Chiral separation of beta-adrenergic antagonists, profen non-steroidal anti-inflammatory drugs and chlorophenoxypropionic acid herbicides using teicoplanin as the chiral selector in capillary liquid chromatography. *J. Chromatogr. A.*, 2005, 1088, 82-93.

[86] Ansell, RJ. Molecularly imprinted polymers for the enantioseparation of chiral drugs. *Adv. Drug Deliv. Rev.*, 2005, 57, 1809-1835.

[87] Nie,Y; Liu, X; Yang, X; Zhao, Z. Recent application of chiral liquid chromatography-tandem mass spectrometric methods for enantiomeric pharmaceutical and biomedical determinations. *J. Chromatogr. Sci.*, 2013, 51, 753-763.

[88] Wan, D; Li, F; Jiang, Z; Yu, L; Guo, X. Chiral Recognition Mechanisms of four β-Blockers by HPLC with Amylose Chiral Stationary Phase. *Iran J. Pharm. Res.*, 2014, 13, 449-457.

[89] Alanazi, AM; Hefnawy, MM; Al-Majed, AA; Al-Suwailem, AK; Kassem, MG; Mostafa, GA; Attia, SM; Khedr, MA. HPLC-fluorescence method for the enantioselective analysis of propranolol in rat serum using immobilized polysaccharide-based chiral stationary phase. *Chirality.*, 2014, 26, 194-199.

[90] Valentová, J; Čižmáriková, R; Bui, TTT; Drake, AF; Hutt, AJ. Enantiomeric resolution of novel aryloxyaminopropanol derivatives with β-adrenoceptor antagonist activity on a derivatised amylose chiral stationary phase. *Chromatographia* 2003, 58, 733-740.

[91] Chen. L; Ma, H; Liu, X; Jiang, SX. Semipreparative enantiomer separation of propranolol hydrochloride by high-performance liquid chromatography using cellulose tris(3,5-dimethylphenylcarbamate) chiral stationary phase. *J. Chromatogr. Sci.*, 2008, 46, 767-771.

[92] Zhang, L; Yu, W; Rong, Y; Guo, X; Ye, J; Shen, Z. Enantiomeric separation of 2-arylpropionic acid nonsteroidal anti-inflammatory drugs and β-blockers by RP-HPLC using amylose chiral stationary phase for enantioselective skin permeation study. *Anal. Methods.*, 2014, 6, 6058-6065.

[93] Ghanem, A; Hoenen, H; Aboul-Enein, HY. Application and comparison of immobilized and coated amylose tris-(3,5-dimethylphenylcarbamate) chiral stationary phases for the enantioselective separation of beta-blockers enantiomers by liquid chromatography. *Talanta.*, 2006, 6, 602-609.

[94] Ilisz, I; Berkecz, R; Péter, A. Retention mechanism of high-performance liquid chromatographic enantioseparation on macrocyclic glycopeptide-based chiral stationary phases. *J. Chromatogr. A.*, 2009, 1216, 1845-1860.

[95] Xia, YQ; Bakhtiar, R; Franklin, RB. Automated online dual-column extraction coupled with teicoplanin stationary phase for simultaneous determination of (*R*)- and (*S*)-propranolol in rat plasma using liquid chromatography-tandem mass spectrometry. *J. Chromatogr. B. Analyt. Technol. Biomed. Life Sci.*, 2003, 788, 317-329.

[96] Nikolai, LN; McClure, EL; Macleod, SL; Wong, CS. Stereoisomer quantification of the beta-blocker drugs atenolol, metoprolol, and propranolol in wastewaters by chiral high-performance liquid chromatography-tandem mass spectrometry. *J. Chromatogr. A*, 2006, 1131, 103-109.

[97] MacLeod, SL; Sudhir, P; Wong, CS. Stereoisomer analysis of wastewater-derived beta-blockers, selective serotonin re-uptake inhibitors, and salbutamol by high-performance liquid chromatography-tandem mass spectrometry. *J. Chromatogr. A*, 2007, 1170, 23-33.

[98] Ribeiro, AR; Santos, LH; Maia. AS; Delerue-Matos, C; Castro, PM; Tiritan, ME. Enantiomeric fraction evaluation of pharmaceuticals in environmental matrices by liquid chromatography-tandem mass spectrometry. *J .Chromatogr. A*, 2014, 1363, 226-235.

[99] Bagnall, JP; Evans, SE; Wort, MT; Lubben, AT; Kasprzyk-Hordern, B. Using chiral liquid chromatography quadrupole time-of-flight mass spectrometry for the analysis of pharmaceuticals and illicit drugs in surface and wastewater at the enantiomeric level. *J. Chromatogr A.*, 2012, 1249, 115-129.

[100] Barbato, F; Carpentiero, C; Grumetto, L; La Rotonda, MI. Enantioselective retention of beta-blocking agents on human serum albumin and alpha 1-acid glycoprotein HPLC columns: relationships with different scales of lipophilicity. *Eur. J. Pharm. Sci.*, 2009, 38, 472-478.

[101] Enquist, M; Hermansson, J. Separation of the enantiomers of beta-receptor blocking agents and other cationic drugs using a CHIRAL-AGP column. Binding properties and characterization of immobilized alpha 1-acid glycoprotein. *J. Chromatogr.*, 1990, 519, 285-298.

[102] Ståhlberg, J; Henriksson, H; Divne. C; Isaksson, R; Pettersson, G; Johansson, G; Jones, TA. Structural basis for enantiomer binding and separation of a common beta-blocker:

crystal structure of cellobiohydrolase Cel7A with bound (*S*)-propranolol at 1.9 A resolution. *J. Mol. Biol.*, 2001, 305, 79-93.

[103] Götmar, G; Fornstedt, T; Andersson, M; Guiochon, G. Influence of the solute hydrophobicity on the enantioselective adsorption of beta-blockers on a cellulase protein used as the chiral selector. *J. Chromatogr., A* 2001, 905, 3-17.

[104] Xuan, H; Hage, DS. Evaluation of a hydrazide-linked alpha1-acid glycoprotein chiral stationary phase: separation of R- and S-propranolol. *J. Sep. Sci.*, 2006, 29, 1412-1422.

[105] Suedee. R; Srichana, T; Martin, GP. Evaluation of matrices containing molecularly imprinted polymers in the enantioselective-controlled delivery of beta-blockers. *J. Control Release.*, 2000, 66, 135-147.

[106] Ansell, RJ. Molecularly imprinted polymers for the enantioseparation of chiral drugs. *Adv. Drug Deliv. Rev.*, 2005, 57, 1809-1835.

[107] Haginaka, J; Sakai, Y. Uniform-sized molecularly imprinted polymer material for (S)-propranolol. *J. Pharm. Biomed. Anal.*, 2000, 22, 899-907.

[108] Guillarme, D; Bonvin, G; Badoud, F; Schappler, J; Rudaz, S; Veuthey, JL. Fast chiral separation of drugs using columns packed with sub-2 microm particles and ultra-high pressure. *Chirality.*, 2010, 22, 320-330.

[109] Gübitz, G; Schmid, MG. Chiral separation by capillary electrochromatography. *Enantiomer.*, 2000, 5, 5-11.

[110] Gübitz, G; Schmid, MG. Advances in chiral separation using capillary electromigration techniques. *Electrophoresis.*, 2007, 28, 114-126.

[111] Scriba, GK. Cyclodextrins in capillary electrophoresis enantioseparations-recent developments and applications. *J. Sep. Sci.*, 2008, 31, 1991-2011.

[112] Tsioupi, DA; Stefan-Vanstaden, RI; Kapnissi-Christodoulou, CP. Chiral selectors in CE: recent developments and applications. *Electrophoresis.* 2013, 34, 178-204.

[113] Chankvetadze, B; Blaschke, G. Enantioseparations using capillary electromigration techniques in nonaqueous buffers. *Electrophoresis.*, 2000, 21, 4159-4178.

[114] Pak, C; Marriott, PJ; Carpenter, PD; Amiet, RG. Enantiomeric separation of propranolol and selected metabolites by using capillary electrophoresis with hydroxypropyl-beta-cyclodextrin as chiral selector. *J. Chromatogr., A* 1998, 793, 357-364.

[115] Hashem, H; Kinzig, M; Jira, T. The effect of achiral calixarenes on chiral separation of propranolol-HCl and brompheniramine maleate in capillary electrophoresis using cyclodextrin as chiral selector. *Pharmazie.*, 2008, 63, 256-262.

[116] Juvancz, Z; Kendrovics, RB; Iványi, R; Szente, L. The role of cyclodextrins in chiral capillary electrophoresis. *Electrophoresis.*, 2008, 29, 1701-1712.

[117] Servais, AC; Rousseau, A; Fillet, M; Lomsadze, K; Salgado, A; Crommen, J; Chankvetadze, B. Capillary electrophoretic and nuclear magnetic resonance studies on the opposite affinity pattern of propranolol enantiomers towards various cyclodextrins. *J. Sep. Sci.*, 2010, 33, 1617-1624.

[118] Matthijs, N; Vander Heyden, Y. Enantiomeric impurity determination in capillary electrophoresis using a highly-sulfated cyclodextrins-based method. *Biomed. Chromatogr.*, 2006, 26, 4116-4126.

[119] Borges, KB; Pupo, MT; Bonato, PS. Enantioselective analysis of propranolol and 4-hydroxypropranolol by CE with application to biotransformation studies employing endophytic fungi. *Electrophoresis.*, 2009, 30, 3910-3917.

[120] Zhu, W; Vigh, G. Enantiomer separations by nonaqueous capillary electrophoresis using octakis(2,3-diacetyl-6-sulfato)-gamma-cyclodextrin. *J. Chromatogr. A.*, 2000, 892, 499-507.

[121] Servais, AC; Rousseau, A; Fillet, M; Lomsadze, K; Salgado, A; Crommen, J; Chankvetadze, B. Separation of propranolol enantiomers by CE using sulfated beta-CD derivatives in aqueous and non-aqueous electrolytes: comparative CE and NMR study. *Electrophoresis.*, 2010, 31, 1467-1474.

[122] Lomsadze, K; Salgado, A; Calvo, E; López, JA; Chankvetadze, B. Comparative NMR and MS studies on the mechanism of enantioseparation of propranolol with heptakis(2,3-diacetyl-6-sulfo)-β-cyclodextrin in capillary electrophoresis with aqueous and non-aqueous electrolytes. *Electrophoresis.*, 2011, 32, 1156-1163.

[123] Feng, Y; Wang, T; Jiang, Z; Chankvetadze, B; Crommen, J. Comparative enantiomer affinity pattern of β-blockers in aqueous and non-aqueous CE using single-component anionic cyclodextrins. *Electrophoresis.*, 2014, 17, doi: 10.1002/elps.201400462. [Epub ahead of print].

[124] Lodén, H; Hedeland, Y; Hedeland, M; Bondesson, U; Pettersson, C. Development of a chiral non-aqueous capillary electrophoretic system using the partial filling technique with UV and mass spectrometric detection. *J. Chromatogr.*, *A* 2003, 986, 143-152.

[125] Hedeland, Y; Haglöf, J; Beronius, P; Pettersson, C. Effect of alkali metal hydroxides on the enantioseparation of amines using di-*O*-isopropylidene-keto-L-gulonic acid as the selector in NACE. *Electrophoresis.*, 2006, 27, 4469-4479.

[126] Wang, LJ; Hu, SQ; Guo, QL; Yang, GL; Chen, XG. Di-n-amyl L-tartrate-boric acid complex chiral selector in situ synthesis and its application in chiral nonaqueous capillary electrophoresis. *J. Chromatogr.*, *A.* 2011, 1218, 1300-1309.

[127] Hödl, H; Krainer, A; Holzmüller, K; Koidl, J; Schmid, MG; Gübitz, G. Chiral separation of sympathomimetics and beta-blockers by ligand-exchange CE using Cu(II) complexes of L-tartaric acid and L-threonine as chiral selectors. *Electrophoresis.*, 2007, 28, 2675-2682.

[128] Xu, H; Yu, X; Chen H. Enantiomeric separation of basic drugs with partially filled serum albumin as chiral selector in capillary electrophoresis. *Anal. Sci.*, 2004, 20, 1409-1413.

[129] Martinez-Pla, JJ; Marrtin-Biosca, Y; Sagrado, S; Villanueva-Camanas, RM; Medina-Hernandez, MJ. Fast enantiomeric separation of propranolol by affinity capillary electrophoresis using human serum albumin as chiral selector: application to quality control of pharmaceuticals. *Anal. Chim. Acta.*, 2004, 507, 171-178.

[130] Yu, T; Du, Y; Chen, B. Evaluation of clarithromycin lactobionate as a novel chiral selector for enantiomeric separation of basic drugs in capillary electrophoresis. *Electrophoresis.*, 2011 , 32, 1898-1905.

[131] Beck, GM; Neau, SH; Holder, AJ; Hemenway, JN. Evaluation of quantitative structure property relationships necessary for enantioresolution with lambda- and sulfobutylether lambda-carrageenan in capillary electrophoresis. *Chirality.*, 2000, 12, 688-696.

[132] Beck, GM; Neau, SH. Optimization of lambda-carrageenan as a chiral selector in capillary electrophoresis separations. *Chirality.*, 2000, 12, 614-620.

[133] Lin, KC; Hsieh, MM; Chang, CW; Lin, EP; Wu, TH. Stacking and separation of aspartic acid enantiomers under discontinuous system by capillary electrophoresis with light-emitting diode-induced fluorescence detection. *Talanta.*, 2010, 82, 1912-1918.

[134] Aturki, Z; D'Orazio, G; Rocco, A; Fanali, S. Advances in the enantioseparation of β-blocker drugs by capillary electromigration techniques. *Electrophoresis.*, 2011, 3, 2602-2628.

[135] Rizvi, SA; Shamsi, SA. Polymeric alkenoxy amino acid surfactants: I. Highly selective class of molecular micelles for chiral separation of beta-blockers. *Electrophoresis.*, 2003, 24, 2514-2526.

[136] Rizvi, SA; Shamsi, SA. Polymeric alkenoxy amino acid surfactants: V. Comparison of carboxylate and sulfate head group polymeric surfactants for enantioseparation in MEKC. *Electrophoresis.*, 2007, 28, 1762-1778.

[137] Akbay, C; Rizvi, SA; Shamsi, SA. Simultaneous enantioseparation and tandem UV-MS detection of eight beta-blockers in micellar electrokinetic chromatography using a chiral molecular micelle. *Anal. Chem.*, 2005, 77, 1672-1683.

[138] Kahle, KA; Foley, JP. Review of aqueous chiral electrokinetic chromatography (EKC) with an emphasis on chiral microemulsion EKC. *Electrophoresis.*, 2007, 28, 2503-2526.

[139] Hu, SQ; Chen, YL; Zhu, HD; Shi, HJ; Yan, N; Chen, XG. Effect of molecular structure of tartrates on chiral recognition of tartrate-boric acid complex chiral selectors in chiral microemulsion electrokinetic chromatography. *J. Chromatogr., A* 2010, 1217, 5529-5535.

[140] Hu, SQ; Lü, WJ; Ma, YH; Hu, Q; Dong, LJ; Chen, XG. Chiral separation of β-blockers by MEEKC using neutral microemulsion: Analysis of separation mechanism and further elucidation of resolution equation. *Electrophoresis.*, 2013, 34, 260-268.

[141] Ma, Y; Zhang, H; Rahman, ZU; Wang, W; Li, X; Chen, H; Chen, X. Sensitive enantioanalysis of β-blockers via field-amplified sample injection combined with water removal in microemulsion electrokinetic chromatography. *Electrophoresis.*, 2014, 35, 2772-2777.

[142] Hsieh, ML; Chau, LK; Hon, YS. Single-step approach for fabrication of vancomycin-bonded silica monolith as chiral stationary phase. *J. Chromatogr., A* 2014, 1358, 208-216.

[143] Chen, Z; Zeng. S; Yao, T. Separation of beta-receptor blockers and analogs by capillary liquid chromatography (CLC) and pressurized capillary electrochromatography (pCEC) using a vancomycin chiral stationary phase column. *Pharmazie.*, 2007, 62, 585-592.

[144] D'Orazio, G; Fanali, S. Coupling capillary electrochromatography with mass spectrometry by using a liquid-junction nano-spray interface. *J. Chromatogr., A* 2010, 1217, 4079-4086.

[145] Dong, X; Dong, J; Ou, J; Zhu, Y; Zou, H. Preparation and evaluation of a vancomycin-immobilized silica monolith as chiral stationary phase for CEC. *Electrophoresis.*, 2007, 28, p. 2606-2612.

[146] Karlsson, C; Wikström, H; Armstrong, DW; Owens PK. Enantioselective reversed-phase and non-aqueous capillary electrochromatography using a teicoplanin chiral stationary phase. *J. Chromatogr., A.* 2000, 897, 349-363.

[147] Chen, X; Qin, F; Liu, Y; Kong, L; Zou, H. Preparation of a positively charged cellulose derivative chiral stationary phase with copolymerization reaction for capillary electrochromatographic separation of enantiomers. *Electrophoresis.*, 2004, 25, 2817-2824.

[148] Mangelings, D; Hardies, N; Maftouh, M; Suteu, C; Massart, DL; Vander Heyden, Y. Enantioseparations of basic and bifunctional pharmaceuticals by capillary electrochromatography using polysaccharide stationary phases. *Electrophoresis.*, 2003, 24, 2567-2576.

[149] Kumar, AP; Park, JH. Fast separations of chiral β-blockers on a cellulose tris(3,5-dimethylphenylcarbamate)-coated zirconia monolithic column by capillary electrochromatography. *J. Chromatogr., A* 2011, 1218, 5369-5373.

[150] Gu, C; Shamsi, SA. Evaluation of a methacrylate-bonded cyclodextrins as a monolithic chiral stationary phase for capillary electrochromatography (CEC)-UV and CEC coupled to mass spectrometry. *Electrophoresis.*, 2011, 32, 2727-2737.

[151] Aturki, Z. Vichi, F; Messina, A; Sinibaldi, M. Indirect resolution of beta-blocker agents by reversed-phase capillary electrochromatography. *Electrophoresis.*, 2004, 25, 607-614.

[152] Guo, WP; Rong, ZB; Li, YH; Fung, YS; Gao, GQ; Cai, ZM. Microfluidic chip capillary electrophoresis coupled with electrochemiluminescence for enantioseparation of racemic drugs using central composite design optimization. *Electrophoresis.*, 2013, 34, 2962-2969.

[153] Belin, GK; Seeger, S. Rapid analysis of serotonin and propranolol using miniaturized CE with deep-UV fluorescence detector. *Electrophoresis.*, 2009, 30, 2565-2571.

[154] Suedee, R; Heard, CHM. Direct resolution of propranolol and bupranolol by thin-layer chromatography using cellulose derivatives as stationary phase. *Chirality.*, 1997, 9, p. 139-144.

[155] Čižmáriková, R; Hroboňová, R; Lehotay, J; Račanská, E; Bruchatá, K. Preparation, pharmacological activity and enantioseparation of [3-(cyklopentyloxymethyl)-4-(hydroxy-3-isopropylaminopropoxy) phenyl]ethanone as potential β-blocker. *Acta Facult. Pharm. Univ. Comen.*, 2005, 52, p. 79-88.

[156] Bhushan, R; Thiongo, GT. Direct enantioseparation of some beta-adrenergic blocking agents using impregnated thin-layer chromatography. *J. Chromatogr. B Biomed. Sci.*, 1998, 708, 330-334.

[157] Bhushan. R, Tanwar, S. Direct TLC resolution of atenolol and propranolol into their enantiomers using three different chiral selectors as impregnating reagents. *Biomed. Chromatogr.*, 2008, 22, 1028-1034.

[158] Čižmáriková, R; Bruchatá K; Pastírová, Z; Lehotay, J; Hroboňová, K. HPLC and TLC enantioseparation of the nitro-positioned aryloxysubstituted aminopropranols. *Pharmazie.*, 2010, 65, 387-388.

[159] Bhushan, R; Tanwar, S. Different approaches of impregnation for resolution of enantiomers of atenolol, propranolol and salbutamol using Cu(II)-L-amino acid complexes for ligand exchange on commercial thin layer chromatographic plates. *J. Chromatogr., A.* 2010, 1217, 1395-1398.

[160] Suedee, R; Srichana, T; Saelim, J; Thavonpibulbut, T. Thin-layer chromatographic separation of chiral drugs on molecularly imprinted chiral stationary phases. *J. Planar. Chromatogr. - Mod. TLC.*, 2001, 4, 194-198.

[161] Suedee, R; Juraiporn Saelim, J; Thavornpibulbut, T; Srichana. T. Chiral determination of various adrenergic drugs by thin-layer chromatography using molecularly imprinted chiral stationary phases prepared with α-agonists. *Analyst.*, 1999, 124, 1003-1009.

[162] Agustian, J; Kamarrudin, AH; Bhatia, S. Single enantiomeric β-blockers - The existing technologies. *Process Biochem.*, 2010, 45, 1587-1604.

[163] Sayyed, IA; Thakur, VV; Nikalje, MD; Dewkar, GK; Kotkar, SP; Sudalai, A. Asymmetric synthesis of aryloxypropanolamines via OsO4-catalyzed asymmetric dihydroxylation. *Tetrahedron.*, 2005, 61, 2831-2838.

[164] Jacobsen, EN. Asymmetric catalysis of epoxide ring-opening reactions. *Acc. Chem. Res.*, 2000, 33, 421-431.

[165] Larrow, JF; Schaus, SE; Jacobsen, EN. Kinetic resolution of terminal epoxides via highly regioselective and enantioselective ring opening with TMSN 3. An efficient, catalytic Route to 1,2-amino alcohols. *J. Am. Chem. Soc.*,1996, 118 , 7420-7421.

[166] Eshghi, H; Porkar Yazdi, H. A facile synthesis of (*S*)-(-)-propranolol. *J. Sci. I. R. Iran.* 2003, 14, 17-19.

[167] Singh, N; Kumar, A; Singh, R. Concise synthesis of (*S*)-(-)-Propranolol: Using acid catalysed kinetic resolution. *J. Chem. Pharm. Res.*, 2012, 4 (12), 5111-5113.

[168] Klunder, MK; Ko, SY; Sharpless, KB. Asymmetric epoxidation od allyl alcohol: efficient routes to homochiral β-adrenergic blocking agents. *J. Org. Chem.*, 1986, 51, 3710-3712.

[169] Inkum, R; Teerawutgulrag, A; Puangsombat, P; Rakariyatham, N. Stereoselective eduction of amino ketone with sodium borohydride in the presence of metal chloride. A simple pathway to S-propranolol. *World Academy of Science, Engineering and Technology*, 2012, 67, 960-963.

[170] Panchgalle, SP; Gore, RG; Chavan, SP; Kalkote, UR. Organocatalytic enantioselective synthesis of β-blockers: (*S*)-propranolol and (*S*)-naftopidil. *Tetrahedron: Asymmetr.*, 2009, 20, 1767-1770.

[171] Veloo, RA; Koomen, GJ. Synthesis of enantiomerically pure (*S*)-(—)-propranolol from sorbitol. *Tetrahedron: Asymmetr.*, 1993, 12, 2401-2404.

[172] Lokhande, MN; Chopade, MU; Bhangare, DN; Nikalje, MD. Asymmetric synthesis of propranolol, naftopidil and (*R*)-monobutyrin using a glycerol desymmetrization strategy. *J. Braz. Chem. Soc.*, 2013, 24 (3), 406-409.

[173] Wunsche, K; Schwaneberg, U; Bornscheuer, UT; Meyer, HH. Chemoenzymatic route to β-blockers via 3-hydroxy esters. *Tetrahedron: Asymmetr.*, 1996, 7, 2017-2022.

[174] Kamal, A; Khanna, GBR; Krishnaji, T; Tekumalla, V; Ramu, R. New chemoenzymatic pathway for β-adrenergic blocking agents. *Tetrahedron: Asymmetr.*, 2005, 16, 1485-1494.

[175] Gihani El, MT; Williams, MJ. Dynamic kinetic resolution. *Curr. Opin. Chem. Biol.*, 1999, 3, p. 11-15.

[176] Pamies, O; Backvall, JE. Dynamic kinetic resolution of β-azido alcohols. An efficient route to chiral aziridines and β-amino alcohols. *J. Org. Chem.*, 2001, 66, 4022-4025.

[177] Yang, W; Xu, JH; Xie, Y; Xu, Y; Zhao, G; Lin, GQ. Asymmetric reduction of ketones by employing Rhodotorula sp. AS2.2241 and synthesis of the β-blocker (*R*)-nifenalol. *Tetrahedron: Asymmetr.*, 2006, 17, 1769-1774.

[178] Kapoor, M; Anand, N; Koul, S; Chimni, SS; Manhas, KS; Raina, C; Parshad, R; Taneja, SC; Qazi, GN. Kinetic resolution of 1-chloro-3-(1-naphthyloxy)-2-propanol, an intermediate in the synthesis of β-adrenergic receptor blockers. *Bioorg. Chem.*, 2003, 31, 259-269.

[179] Čižmáriková, R; Valentová, J; Hutt, AJ; Sedláková, S. Beta-adrenergic blockers- a group of chiral drugs: Stereoselective synthesis of β-blockers. *Čes. Slov. Farm.*, 2005, 5, 201-206 [in slovak].

[180] Jung, ME; Shaw, TJ. Total synthesis of *(R)*- glycerol acetonide and the antiepileptic and hypotensive drug (-)-γ-amino-β-hydroxybutyric acid (GABOOB): use of vitamin C as a chiral starting material. *J. Am. Chem. Soc.*, 1980, 102, 6304-6311.

[181] Feng, A; Chen, Y; Cheng, Y. Asymmetric synthesis of (2*S*)-propranolol using D-mannitol. *J. Chem. Pharm. Res.*, 2013, 5, 349-352.

[182] Kan, K; Miyama, A; Hamaguchi, S; Ohashi, T; Watanabe, K. Synthesis of (*S*)-β-blockers from (*S*)-5-hydroxymethyl-3-tert butyl-2-oxazolidinone or (*S*)-5-hydroxymethyl-3-isopropyl-2-oxazolidinone. *J. Agric. Chem.*, 1985, 49, 207-210.

[183] Viegas, RMC; Afonso, CAM; Crespo, JG; Coelhoso, IM. Modelling of the enantio-selective extraction of propranolol in biphasic system. *Separ. Purif. Tech.*, 2007, 53, 224-234.

[184] Viegas RMC; Afonso, CAM; Crespo, JG; Coelhoso, IM. Racemic resolution of propranolol in membrane contractors: Modelling and process optimisation. *J. Membr. Sci.*, 2007, 305, 203-214.

[185] Krause, HW; Schmidt, U; Foken, H. Preparation of optically active propranolol analogues. *Pharmazie*, 1992, 47, 838-841.

Index

A

D

E

F

G

H

I

K

L

O

P

Q

R

T

U

V

W

X

Y

Z